Breaking the Age Barrier

Breaking the Age Barrier

HELEN FRANKS

Ulysses Press Berkeley, CA

1996

Published by: Ulysses Press
   P.O. Box 3440
   Berkeley, CA 94703-3440

Library of Congress Catalog Card Number: 95-61135

ISBN: 1-56975-044-0

First published as *Getting Older—Slowly: Your Guide to Successful Ageing* by Rosendale Press

Printed in the USA by R.R. Donnelley & Sons

10 9 8 7 6 5 4 3 2 1

Editorial and production: Leslie Henriques, Joanna Pearlman, Ellen Nidy,
  Claire Chun, Lee Micheaux, Toby Bielawski
Cover Design: The Visual Group
Front cover photograph: Catherine Gockley/Superstock
Indexer: Sayre Van Young

Distributed in the United States by Publishers Group West and in Canada by Raincoast Books.

I don't believe in aging. I believe in forever altering one's aspect to the sun.

—Virginia Woolf

Table of Contents

Chapter 3: The Challenge of Staying Healthy

Chapter 4: The Challenge of Looking Good

Chapter 5: The Brain Challenge

Chapter 6: The Lifestyle Challenge

Bibliography

Index

Acknowledgements

Many individuals and organizations have supplied information for this book, for which I am extremely grateful. My special thanks go to the following: Age Concern, Institute of Alcohol Studies, American Longevity Research Institute, Carol Bateman of the Royal Free Hospital, British Geriatric Society, British Heart Foundation, Centre for Policy on Ageing, the Food Commission, Dr. John Faulkner of the University of Michigan Institute of Gerontology, Dr. Donald Gould, Gallup Polls, Imperial Cancer Research Foundation, Dee Knapp, the MacArthur Foundation Network on Successful Midlife Development, Dr. Edward Masoro of the University of Texas Aging Research and Education Center, Medical Resource Service (U.K.), Medical Resource Service (U.S.), National Institute on Aging, Bethesda, Elizabeth Nelson, Research Into Ageing, Ray Rice of the Fish Foundation, Dr. Judith Rodin of the MacArthur Foundation Network on Health and Behavior, Dr. Alice Rossi of the Midmac project, Dr. John Rowe of the MacArthur Foundation Network on Successful Aging, Dawn Skelton, Vitamin E Information Service, and last but not least Rebecca Trup who put everything into rational order.

Helen Franks

Introduction

AGING—A NEW AGENDA

Is it an illusion, or is it really true that people are staying younger longer? A few decades ago, we thought senior citizens were tired, elderly people who sat on park benches feeding the pigeons. Now we find that they travel to exotic places, go to aerobics classes, take courses in philosophy, join activist groups and even bungee jump.

Researchers speak of the "young elderly" or "third agers," people up to about 75 who are mentally and physically more vital than those of a similar age just a few decades ago. They say that the idea of aging as a continuous decline is outdated. In a study published in 1992, it was found that many functions are relatively unchanged by the age of 75 years, while verbal ability and short-term memory showed little deterioration in healthy individuals at 85.

Most important of all, many of the conditions we associate with aging, such as high cholesterol levels, stroke, heart disease and cancer, are not the inevitable consequences of getting old. In recent years, there has been a substantial decrease in the incidence of stroke, as well as a decrease in deaths from heart disease. Changes in diet, smoking and physical activity are having such a dramatic effect that scientists expect this will lead to an average life expectancy of 85 years by the year 2000.

The present average life expectancy at birth in developed countries is around 78 years for women and 72 years for men. If we survive to the age of 50, we can expect to go on to the age of 81 for women, 76 for men. Life expectancy has been slowly rising since the 1970s, and more of us can expect to see our hundredth birthday. In 1952 the Queen of England sent 200 telegrams to centenarians across the realm; in 1991 she sent 2689.

Even so, the maximum number of years humans can live is limited to around 115. Don't believe all you hear about people living to 150 in isolated populations with simple lifestyles. Wherever written birth records have been consulted, it has been found that the locals have gone in for a certain amount of age exaggeration, no doubt to please enthusiastic anthropologists. The truth is that the people of Vilcabamba, Ecuador, the Hunza of Pakistan and those in Abkhazia, Russia, all of whom claim sensational longevity, actually have the same proportion of people over 90 years old as is found in the United States.

This could change within our lifetimes. Scientists are beginning to make startling predictions about longevity in humans, based on research with other species. The fruit fly, for instance, given a certain amount of gene manipulation, can live to the equivalent of 150 human years. The Human Genome Project, which is well on its way to identifying all genes, will change the way diseases are predicted and treated. Genes specifically connected with aging will provide new kinds of therapies. Biomarkers, clinical tests that provide measurement of the aging status, will provide accurate clinical measurement of a person's aging status. Research into hormones, closely linked with genetic findings, points the way to a cocktail of rejuvenating body chemicals and replacement hormones by about the year 2010, which could increase our average life span to 115.

Our present and immediate future is no less dramatic. The proportion of the population over the age of 65 is rising. In the United States, the current 26 million people over 65 represent 11 percent of the population; by the year 2030 it will be 55 million and 18 percent.

The reason for these changes is not only that we are living longer. It is also that we are having fewer babies. In the mid-19th century we had high birth rates and high death rates. By the early to mid-20th century we had high birth rates and low death rates, with a drop in babies dying in infancy and women dying in childbirth. Now we have a new shape for what is called the age pyramid, with low birth rates making the base of the pyramid slimmer in proportion to the number of people growing older.

For those of us with old age on the horizon, the age we want to live to—whether it's 115, 150 or even 85—is less important than *how* we want to live. We don't want extra years filled with the diseases associated with old age. Heart disease is still a leading cause of death in most developed countries. Alzheimer's disease currently affects four million Americans. Hip fractures continue to be a serious threat largely due to osteoporosis in women, especially in those who are not physically active and who have had a low calcium diet. Poverty in western societies is associated with chronic illness in middle and old age, and higher death rates.

Some of the factors contributing to later-life disability are out of our hands. We must look to science to manipulate our genes and to government policies to help keep us financially above water, give us work flexibility, provide opportunities for continued learning through adult education classes and encourage us to network as volunteers and caregivers.

But there is much that we can do ourselves to make our future bright. A great deal of it you will find in this book.

CHAPTER ONE

The Fitness Challenge

EXERCISE CAN CHANGE
THE WAY YOU GROW OLD

I had watched my neighbor getting more and more frail. She was in her late 80s and finally accepted that she needed some nursing assistance. She could no longer get herself out of the bath, and her doctor arranged for a nurse to come in twice a week to assist her. My neighbor, a very independent woman, resisted the proposal vigorously. Neither doctor nor nurse suggested another possibility: that she might be given exercises to strengthen her weakened muscles.

EXERCISE AT ANY AGE

Exercises at 80-something may sound a little ambitious, but the truth is that exercise at *any* age can strengthen muscles. Started in midlife and kept up regularly, it can postpone loss of independence into very old age. Experts today agree that it is the one certain aid to fitness and longevity. In the past few years, the evidence has been mounting steadily.

The 30-year Harvard Alumni Health Study of 10,000 men shows that those who have been regularly using up 2000 calories a week in aerobic activity add 2.5 years to their life expectancy. Other findings in this study have shown that moderate aerobic exercise lowers cholesterol, keeps blood pressure down and helps reduce diabetes and hardening of the arteries. And there's the possibility that burning 1000 calories a week or more can halve the risk of colon cancer. Current investigations are covering the possible role of exercise as a prevention for breast cancer.

Walkng 20 minutes three times a week retards aging in middle-aged women, according to another study. When the exercisers, aged from 46 to 50, were compared with nonexercisers over a three-year span, the latter increased in weight, and had elevated blood pressure and blood lipids (fat levels which put them in danger of heart disease), whereas the exercisers had safe cholesterol levels, normal blood pressure and had put on only very small amounts of weight.

Postmenopausal women can maintain and even increase their bone density through exercise. When 53 women, postmenopausal for one to ten years, followed a weight-training exercise regime three times a week for up to 18 months, they retained or gained bone density in the lower back and hip-thigh area at a time of life when they would have been expected to show decline.

And a piece of evidence that could cheer my neighbor comes from a Boston nursing home where a geriatrician persuaded ten people to take up weightlifting and found they more than doubled their muscle power. The volunteers, aged from 86 to 96, most with a history of falls and use of a cane or a walker, lifted weights three times a week for up to 20 minutes over a period of eight weeks. Some of them ended up with a mind-boggling 174 percent increase in leg muscle strength and a 9 percent gain in muscle size, and were able to give up their canes and walkers in the bargain.

Exercise is the one lifestyle factor most important to health—even more significant than not smoking. Among a random selection of nearly 1000 retired people over 65 who were studied for a period of five years, those who exercised enjoyed better health and greater strength than nonexercisers, regardless of sex, socioeconomic status, body weight, age or smoking habits.

When 87 healthy volunteers aged from 60 to 81 were randomly allocated a weekly aerobics class or a health education group, both increased their activity levels, lowered their blood pressure and reported a more positive mental outlook, too. At the end of the five-month study, the exercisers also achieved greater knee and spine flexibility and back strength.

And so it goes. Exercise can also make you feel sexy, may reduce moderate depression, speed up reaction time, improve mental alertness and boost the immune system, making you more resistant to colds or flu.

WHAT HAPPENS IF YOU DON'T EXERCISE

The information on this is expanding, too. If you don't exercise after about the age of 25, you begin to lose flexibility and strength. By the time you're an over-50 nonexerciser, you can expect joint stiffness, reduced muscle mass, lower bone density and diminished lung capacity.

HOW MUCH MUSCLE POWERS GOES

Dawn Skelton, when working at the Human Performance Laboratory at the Royal Free Hospital in London, measured functional ability in men and women aged from 65 to 85 years and found that muscle strength was lost at the rate of about 2 percent a year and lower limb power at 3.5 percent a year in people who did not exercise regularly. Over a lifetime, say between the ages of 30 and 80, muscle strength diminishes by 30 percent in the arms and 40 percent in the legs and back.

These kinds of losses mean that when an 80 year old stumbles, he or she is unlikely to stop that stumble from becoming a fall, with consequences like potentially fatal hip fractures. (It's not the fracture that kills, but the immobility that can lead to other complications such as pneumonia.)

Everyday inactivity in old age exposes us to another danger, hypothermia, or low body temperature, a risk that Skelton demonstrated with 18 young-adult volunteers. The unlucky 18 were immersed in cold water to observe the effect on their muscle power, which was reduced, temporarily, by 25 percent. The muscle cooling was near to that expected in immobile elderly people in underheated homes, and you need little imagination to predict the aftereffect. (One study of falls among women aged 70-plus showed that there were more falls in winter. Not outdoors though. The cause was thought to be due to the women becoming less active, spending more time inside their homes.)

Loss of muscle power does more than increase the risk of falling as we age. It makes climbing stairs, especially steep ones, an increasing strain; it means we struggle out of low chairs by depending heavily on the arm supports, and have difficulty getting up from toilet seats; it means we lose handgrip strength so we can't carry heavy shopping bags or open jars.

The greater muscle power of men at all ages gives them a certain advantage over women. Skelton compared performance in 50 men and 50 women aged from 65 to 89 and found that 20 percent of the men over 85, but no woman over 80, could manage to step up a height of 20 inches. All the men could manage 16 inches, but only a few women over 85 could do so. Many public buses have a 12- to 15-inch step up from the street. Fortunately, muscle power can be reclaimed in dramatic amounts, as the Boston weightlifting trial demonstrates. That study also provided evidence of growth of new muscle fibers. Loss of muscle power is now known to be due to a diminishing of muscle fibers.

CHANGES IN LUNG CAPACITY

Lungs become stiffer and less elastic with age, so we can't breathe in and blow out as much air as in our younger days. Maximum breathing capacity may decline by about 40 percent between the ages of 20 and 70. This means we have to work harder to breathe in more oxygen as we age. Poorer air exchange and weaker lung power allow bacteria to build up more easily in the lungs and make older people more vulnerable to chest infections. Research into diminished lung power and aging is still in its infancy, but there's some evidence to suggest that age is not the total explanation. Height may also be a factor. But lack of sufficient exercise could also be important. Alison McConnell, a university lecturer in human biology, has devised "trainer devices" to redevelop respiratory muscles in the elderly. In a pilot study she observed a group of volunteers aged 62 to 82 using her device daily for six weeks, at the end of which the volunteers demonstrated increased lung function. A control group using dummy devices showed no improvement. Since production costs would be moderate, if further studies prove equally successful, the device could one day be made widely available.

LOSS OF BONE

Menopause is a time of increased aging for women in terms of loss of bone density. A gradual loss of bone with age is common to everyone, but in some women the loss accelerates to 2 to 3 percent a year at the onset of menopause. By the age of 70, a third of a woman's bone mineral mass may have disappeared. This development, called osteoporosis, is said to affect one woman in four and can result in brittle bones and fractures of the hip, leg or arm, or painful compression of the vertebrae. Though hormone replacement therapy (HRT) and other drugs taken after menopause can arrest bone loss or even replace bone, the effect of exercise on muscle power and coordination as well as bone strengthening remains extremely important. See Chapter Three for more on menopause.

THE VO MAX FACTOR

Age-related changes associated with inactivity are now being measured in terms of oxygen replacement. Lack of exercise reduces the body's ability to absorb oxygen from the atmosphere and into the bloodstream and body tissues. The capacity for oxygen absorption can be measured scientifically and is known as VO max (the V is for volume, the O for oxygen converted into carbon dioxide by the body in one minute during maximum physical exertion). Peak age for VO max is around 20, when heart, lungs and muscles are at top capacity. From around 30 there is a slow decline closely associated with physical deterioration and aging. Scientists calculate that nonexercisers reach minimum VO max levels for survival somewhere between the ages of 60 and 90. The physically active can slow the decline and can add about 10 years to their chances of survival.

Based on current knowledge, a nonexerciser between the ages of 50 and 60 can lose around 20 percent of muscle strength, 35 percent of leg and back power and, if a postmenopausal woman, up to 30 percent of bone density. And then there's the 40 percent decline in lung power between the ages of 20 and 70 and the vital VO max oxygen capacity.

Some weakening is inevitable with age—you can't actually stop the clock. In sports, peak-performance ages range from the late teens for swimming, to the mid-20s for running events and tennis, the late 20s for baseball, and the early 30s for golf. After that, a gradual decline is expected. The same will occur in nonathletes, but in every age group research has shown that the decline can be slowed down by regular exercise.

THE RIGHT KINDS OF EXERCISE

Walking, weightlifting, jogging—all of these have shown how they can postpone the aging process. If you exercise your heart and lungs you maintain aerobic power; if you work your muscles and joints you retain or regain body strength and bone thickness; if you stretch, you stay flexible. Basically, that's all there is to it. Pick a mixture of aerobics, muscle and bone strengtheners and stretches, and do them for a minimum total of three hours a week. The important thing is to do them regularly. (Note: Be sure to consult your doctor before beginning any exercise program.)

AEROBICS

Aerobics are activities that get the heart pumping fast. In other words, if you don't get out of breath you're not engaging in an aerobic activity. The point of the exercise is to raise the pulse (see page 19 to find out how you can check your pulse).

Walking is aerobic when you get a little winded, not when you do a gentle stroll. You don't have to get so winded that you're gasping for air, but enough to make it a bit difficult to keep a conversation without some heavy breathing. An easy test: You should be able to talk, but not sing. Jogging, swimming, cycling, fast dancing and tennis all count as aerobics.

How often to do them: Up to one hour three times a week. It is best to have a day's rest in between. Less than 15 minutes of a good workout will bring no benefit; more than 40 minutes of fast action does little extra. A good half-hour of strenuous activity plus warm-up and cool-down are best. Never exercise to the point of exhaustion, and if you're 50-plus and new to it, talk to your doctor first.

MUSCLE STRENGTHENERS AND BONE BOOSTERS

These work on arms, shoulders, abdominals, hips and buttocks, and legs. Working the muscles maintains the number of fibers—a reduction in the number of fibers means muscles weaken. The movements also create pressure on bones and helps retain their density—important for postmenopausal women to reduce the chance of osteoporosis. You can try weight-training classes or work out at home with bottles and cans, which is best done by following a book, video or cassette. Or follow an exercise regime designed to increase bone density and prevent osteoporosis—it will work on muscles, too. Hatha yoga also provides bone-impact and muscle-strengthening exercises.

How often to do them: A minimum of 20 minutes three times a week, again working hard but not to the point of pain or discomfort. Hatha yoga offers stretch and flexibility as well as strength. It's best if you go to a class and work up strength gradually under supervision.

STRETCH EXERCISES

These work on neck, back, arms, legs and hips. If you don't stretch, muscles get shorter and tighter, resulting in stiffness and reduced mobility. Yoga is also effective, and there are remedial yoga classes for the very stiff. You can find a variety of stretch routines in classes and from books, videos and cassettes. Stretching can be incorporated into the warm-up and cool-down when doing aerobics. Make special time for them if you rely on brisk walking as your aerobic exercise.

How often to do them: Five minutes a day, three times a week minimum. If you work at a desk or sit still a great deal, get up after an hour and take a few minutes off for a mini-stretch session before sitting again. Stretch exercises lying flat on the bed are one way to get started if you're very stiff.

PUTTING THE RECORD RIGHT—
SOME MYTHS AND FACTS ABOUT EXERCISE

Myth: Exercise only does you good if it hurts.

Going for the burn is old hat. It can put a strain on the heart and can damage muscles and joints. A gentle start, building up to greater endurance over weeks and months is the modern approach to sports and exercise. Never work yourself to the point of exhaustion—not only do you risk injury, but you're not making yourself fitter by overreaching your capacity. More than three hours of exercise a week does not produce increasing health advantages.

Myth: Those suffering from joint pain and stiffness shouldn't exercise.

Only 7 percent of people over 50 say they never suffer from joint pain and stiffness. About half of those who do get the pains believe, quite mistakenly, that they should not exercise.

Fact: Exercise increases your appetite if you do it only occasionally.

Exercise regularly and the reverse is true. Appetite and hunger increase when blood sugar plummets, but regular exercise helps keep blood sugar stable and appetite can actually decrease.

Myth: Exercise requires you to eat more protein.

Yet another fallacy. However, some potassium and magnesium are lost in perspiration, and magnesium, chromium and zinc are excreted in greater amounts following exercise. Also, there are increased carbohydrate needs for anyone who is physically active. Replace potassium within a few hours of a workout by eating oranges, tomatoes, bananas, dried fruit or nuts. There's magnesium in nuts, too, and also in meat, fish, dried peas and beans, grains, dark leafy vegetables and milk. Some of these foods contain iron, which may also be lost through excessive exercise. Chromium and zinc sources are whole-grain breads, cereals, meat and vegetables. Carbohydrates are needed to provide energy, and you get them from pasta, potatoes, bread, cereals and rice. Finally, ensure you get vitamin C by eating fruit and green vegetables.

Myth: High-intensity exercise is more effective than lower-intensity exercise, and both give better results in a class than working out at home.

True or false? Three groups of previously sedentary northern California men and women, aged 50 to 65, were compared after a year of regular exercising. One group did high-intensity exercise in a class, the second did high-intensity at home, the third did low-intensity exercise at home. A fourth group was merely assessed as a control. The results? All three exercising groups, but not the control group, improved significantly in fitness, whether on high- or low-intensity programs, in a class or at home.

Fact: Sweating becomes less efficient as a cooling device as we get older.

A man of 50 sweats more slowly than a man of 20, and does so mainly after a bout of exercising rather than during it. (Unfortunately, women don't seem to have been similarly investigated—maybe an echo of old ideas about ladies "glowing" rather than sweating?)

Fact: The warm-up is not just a tiresome idea thought up by overly cautious doctors.

If you don't warm up before exercising, you can overstretch muscles, damage joints and experience strains and pains. More importantly, you put too great a strain on the heart, which like any other complex piece of machinery (such as cars, computers or musical instruments) needs a gradual tune-up before it works at full capacity (see page 19).

Myth: Exercise wears you out.

On the contrary, it increases energy, including that of the sexual variety. Around 31 percent of 8000 Los Angeles women said they had more frequent sex once they began an exercise program; 40 percent noted an increase in arousal and 25 percent experienced an increase in ability to reach orgasm. All this for a minimum of three hours a week of moderate tennis, walking, swimming or cycling. When a group of aerobic-exercising 40- to 50-year-old men kept a diary of their sexual activity for the University of California at San Diego, they reported showing increased interest and more frequent intercourse—over three times a week compared to over twice before they exercised. The aerobics were in the form of 40 minutes jogging or trampoline-jumping five days a week, plus stretch and warm-up exercises. The 78 men were compared with a group of moderate-paced walkers, who failed to show similar gains.

Fact: That old saying "if you don't use it, you lose it" is all too true.

When exercisers who have participated in trials are retested several months after the completion of the study, they show a return-to-before in their physical condition if they haven't continued the exercise. Yes, you can take some time off, but you need to exercise regularly for at least nine months a year to retain the advantages. And it's not a case of taking three months off every year, merely the odd week here and there.

WHAT'S STOPPING YOU

Only about 8 percent of the population in the United States exercises regularly. A report from the Carnegie Trust, focusing on "third agers" (defined as those between 50 and 74) estimates that one-third of men and well over one-half of all women over 65 cannot get up from a chair without using their arms for support. Nearly all women over 55 could not walk up a gentle slope of three degrees at three miles an hour, and walking on a flat surface at the same pace is impossible for half of all women aged 55-plus. There are many reasons for this evidence of inactivity in older people, and they do not all have to do with laziness or even personal disinclination.

One problem with exercise is that you don't see immediate results. On the contrary, your first effort may show up a lack of strength and cause muscle aches. The shift in lifestyle requires effort, perhaps boring or seemingly unrewarding effort, and it may be much easier to ignore the whole business. Also, the mentally aware and active may kid themselves that they are as agile in body as they are in mind.

IT'S NEVER TOO LATE TO START EXERCISING

Mrs. Madge Sharples gave up running the London Marathon at the age of 73. She ran in her first marathon when she was 64 and only stopped because the wear and tear became too much: "I was beginning to feel pain in my good knee." She didn't think about keeping fit when she was younger. Five pregnancies and living abroad with a husband in the diplomatic service kept her too busy. Her life as an exerciser began at the age of 62 with yoga, and went on from there to include weightlifting, body building and swimming.

The medical profession, although now embracing the "E" word in a big way, has a lot to answer for in reinforcing negative attitudes. Even within the last 20 years, many doctors have been of the opinion that fitness potential was mainly based on the genes you were born with, so that if you deteriorated with age there was nothing you could do about it. They said that exercise would damage the heart and wear out bones and joints. Weight training, or indeed any strength-testing activity, was seen as at best useless and at worst dangerous for the elderly, and doctors gave many of their patients the idea that what they really "deserved" was a good rest. The middle-aged to old-aged person who asked for medical clearance before, say, starting to jog, was likely to be indulged as a slight eccentric, a health freak, and at best encouraged with half-hearted enthusiasm.

Today, more doctors are concerned with instilling in their patients the importance of preventive medicine through a healthy lifestyle, but even they may discriminate. A report in 1991 showed that doctors in general practice gave health education advice less often to patients in lower socioeconomic groups than they did to higher socioeconomic groups, and also gave less advice to women than to men. The doctors in the report perceived that a majority of their patients would benefit from lifestyle changes, but the patients themselves, without the necessary guidance, stuck to the traditional passive role, convinced that their problems were due less to lifestyle factors than to external ones over which they had little control.

KEEP ACTIVE

When reading, watching television or working at a computer, never sit for longer than an hour. Get up, stretch and move about the room. Take a few deep breaths and pull your shoulders back and down. Check that they stay that way and sit or stand without hollowing your back.

FOURTEEN EXCUSES FOR NOT EXCERCISING

1. "My doctor said I should be careful."

If your doctor really did say this, ask him or her to explain exactly why. There may be a very good medical reason. It may be important, for instance, that you don't put any pressure on joints if you suffer from severe osteoporosis or osteoarthritis. However, it is also possible that the caution was linked to a temporary medical condition, perhaps when you were convalescing. After illness or an operation, some resting time may be necessary. Always check with your doctor before resuming exercise after an illness. See "Playing Safe—Recognizing and Avoiding Risks," in this chapter for more details on the risks involved in exercising.

2. "I was terrible at games at school, and I don't want to make a fool of myself now."

This attitude has been traditional among girls, who knew they could get out of games at school when they had their period, and who never gained the confidence or the taste for a sport in adult life. Today young women may be more liberated, but still appear to be inactive. Both boys and girls are being seduced by television and computer games. A survey in 1993 showed that two out of three schoolchildren aged from 11 to 14 failed to get enough exercise, with girls less likely than boys. Other reports comparing children in the United Kingdom and Senegal suggest that low levels of physical activity among 11 to 16 year olds are the norm, with little evidence of a raised heart rate in day-to-day life. The Senegalese, by the way, took part in many rural activities such as drawing water, pounding grain, leading donkeys and herding cattle, yet experienced fewer periods of intense physical activity than did the western children. Habits in early life set people up for later, and there's evidence that those who exercise in their youth are more likely to continue or resume exercise in later years. The Allied Dunbar National Fitness Survey of nearly 4500 adults in 1990 showed that 25 percent of those active when aged 14 to 19 years were still active at the time of the survey. Only 2 percent of those who had been inactive in their teens were currently active. Personality in young adulthood can predict the amount of exercise engaged in 40 years later, claims another piece of research. Frequent exercisers in their youth were likely to be vital, well-adjusted individuals with political or practical interests; minimal exercisers were likely to be sensitive, anxious individuals with scientific or aesthetic interests, says Paula Schnurr, summing up a long-term study of Harvard graduates. The data did not show greatly reduced activity by late middle age, perhaps because this was a privileged group with access to superior health care. The inference was that personality counts as much as an athletic physique.

3. *"I can't go to a class until I've lost weight. I'd look terrible in a leotard."*

Looking terrible is a fear that haunts most women, whatever their appearance. Many exercise for the sake of appearance rather than for enjoyment, and can easily get into the double bind of not wanting to join a class till they feel sufficiently confident about their bodies. Overweight teenagers go out of their way to be excused from sports. Girls in early adolescence may gain "puppy fat" and be very self-conscious of their developing bodies. The habit of self-consciousness is reinforced by a lifetime of invidious comparisons and stereotyped yardsticks of perfection. It can take guts and confidence to join a class. For anyone not strong on either of these things, the solution is to choose something noncompetitive, like yoga or stretch dance, in a nonglitzy setting, and wear something loose and nonclingy like a baggy T-shirt and sweatpants.

4. "I don't have time to fit in exercise."

Are you really so busy, or so disorganized, or perhaps so fearful of commitment? Finding time and space for a new, regular activity can require an extraordinary amount of mental energy. It is only too easy to prevaricate, dread the potential "burden" and in fact expend quite a lot of stressful and unproductive energy through avoidance. Once launched into a project, it can quickly become a routine part of life and a source of satisfaction. But the first thing to do is to make a decision and then put it into action.

5. "I used to play a lot of sports, but I suffered an injury."

Sometimes an athletic person who sustains an injury or finds that a sport is too exhausting simply gives up. The energetic racquetball player, for instance, may suffer a sports injury and decide that enough is enough at the age of 40 or 50 or 60. Playing a less difficult game, or dropping down to one session a week, or taking up a gentler sport—golf, bowling, walking—are better solutions than giving up altogether.

6. "I hate the way people try to bully you into exercising."

Stubborn, eh? Don't like anyone telling you what to do? Just remember that you are making your own choices, and there is no point in shooting yourself in the foot in order to thwart others. You can choose to be resistant to "authority," or tell yourself that authority doesn't matter. And who are these bullying people anyway? Since they are at least partly in your own head, you can substitute some purposeful decisions that put you in charge of what you want to do with your life, even if you do in the end decide to be a couch potato.

7. *"I don't need to exercise, I'm on my feet all day anyway."*

This attitude is shared by those who do lots of housework, or who perceive themselves as being physically active in their work, and office workers who have to take a longish walk to the bus stop. They may be totally wrong. Housework, a short stroll, or even painting or decorating, are unlikely to provide sufficient sustained exercise that raises the heart rate. In the Allied Dunbar National Fitness Survey, 80 percent of men and women of all ages believed themselves to be fit or believed that they did enough exercise to keep fit. In fact, around eight out of ten fell below the amount of activity necessary to achieve a health benefit. Echoing the Carnegie survey findings, this survey found that over 50 percent of women aged 55 plus could not walk on level ground at three miles per hour. And 30 percent of men and 50 percent of women aged 65 to 74 did not have sufficient muscle strength to lift half their body weight—which is another way of saying that they couldn't rise from their chair without using their arms.

8. *"I did go to classes, but they're difficult to get to/the hall is drafty and dirty/I didn't like the teacher."*

Excuses, excuses. Arrange to go with a friend and get a lift. Find somewhere else. Try again, your first impressions may have been wrong.

9. *"I find all this emphasis on exercise infantile and moralistic—it's just an escape from facing the inevitable."*

Exercise does not promise immortality. You probably *will* get stiffer, and certainly weaker, with age. But being fatalistic is no more worthy than being moralistic or escapist.

10. *"My parents never exercised, and they seemed okay in old age."*

There may be something in this, though no one really knows whether good genes make you age better. You don't know that you will age as your parents did, and anyway, how can you be sure they didn't hide some of their infirmities, or their secret exercise sessions, from you?

The oldest person to climb Mount Everest was a 60-year-old Venezuelan violin maker, who achieved the feat in October 1993. This beat the record of an American who climbed the mountain in 1985 when he was 55.

11. "I tried to do some exercise, but I ached for days afterward."

There is a difference between "healthy" pain after exercising and unhealthy pain. Muscles can ache because they are being used after months or years of disuse, and if you ache a lot after exercise, then you were probably working too fast. A few days off and you can resume with greater moderation.

Some muscle ache is a sign that you are working well, so you can look on it as positive rather than negative. You do have to make an effort, feel some exertion and experience some breathlessness when exercising and, again, you can view that as positive. When you see a hill ahead, think "good, that will challenge me more than walking on level ground" instead of dreading the slight discomfort. You get to know your body through testing it a little and going through a moderate discomfort barrier, recognizing the difference between true pain that puts a strain on the body and physical effort that tests your strength. One of the advantages of working out in a class with a qualified teacher is that you can question and get immediate feedback. Then you quickly learn when, say, your knee feels an unhealthy strain or your lower back aches in a damaging way. Confidence in one's body comes with the experience of using it, and at times testing it.

12. "I suffer from back pain. I know instinctively that any strain could be damaging."

Back pain is often self-reinforcing, through fear of pain. Instead of testing the waters as you get back to normal after an injury, you may find yourself increasingly self-protective, avoiding certain movements in case of pain. This self-imposed restriction creates further stiffness that can quickly become chronic. Remember, muscles, joints and bones deteriorate with disuse, so exertion becomes progressively difficult. Self-protection can also stem from self-pity—you're too delicate to be put through all the grueling work which some nasty people are trying to force on you.

13. *"It would never work for me."*

This smacks of self-pity too. After making every other excuse you can think of, you're down to the deepest negative attitude, total resignation. Nonexercisers are notorious for underestimating their physical capability. But the big question here is how would you expect it not to work for you? Exercise is inevitably linked with appearance, so for some it could signify a desire, or fear, to re-enter the sexual game. Or it could hold the promise of a lifting of spirits. Anyone who is depressed might well fear the potential disappointment. Maybe other kinds of help are needed.

14. *"I find exercising boring."*

There are many different kinds of exercise. Choose something you don't find boring. See the next section.

GETTING STARTED AND STAYING WITH IT

Various subtle restrictions and stereotypes surround the way we choose exercise. One survey of men and women over 65 showed that the men went for outdoor and leisure activities while the women felt limited by tradition to indoor activity. The fear of rape in secluded areas of parks and open spaces may deter many women who would like to walk or jog, especially if they have to do it alone. Weight training, which is an excellent way to strengthen bones and prevent osteoporosis, may be associated in the minds of some women with developing large muscles (not true if moderate weights are used). Yoga may appear to be a soft option for men, even though one of the most popular methods has been developed by a man. Dancing may be thought of as too "youth oriented" by some older women.

Many people are put off by the idea of physical exercise because they don't see themselves as sporty types, think they are uncoordinated, or don't like competitive sports. Or they don't want to invest in expensive equipment.

NARROWING THE CHOICES

It's important to find activities that are enjoyable and that fit into your lifestyle. You can narrow down the choices by asking yourself a few questions:

- Do you prefer noncompetitive activity?

- Do you mind being outdoors in colder weather? Do you want to exercise alone or in a group?

- Are you happy with strangers or do you want to exercise with a partner or friend?

- Do you want to meet new friends?

- Which is more important to you—fun or concentration?

- Do you work best with rhythm and music?

- Do you want aerobics that put the least stress on your back?

- Do you want to choose something with minimum financial outlay?

Pick and choose from dancing, swimming, jogging, walking, cycling, skipping, trampoline jumping, rowing, weight training, playing tennis or other ball games, using exercise bicycles, rowing machines, treadmills in a gym or at home, or using a cassette or video workout at home.

When you first try a sport or activity, don't push yourself too hard, and don't expect too much. You may be amazed by your unexpected abilities, but if you find the going hard, remember that the greatest discouragement can come in the first attempts. Stick with it and you may well be pleasantly surprised within days or weeks.

Keep regular spaces in your diary for your exercise routine, three sessions a week, and remember to include a warm-up, cool-down and stretching. If you're working out at home alone, arrange the timing of your exercise with a friend, so you can compare afterward. If you like variety, choose several different activities.

BEFORE YOU START

Allow two hours after eating a snack, or four hours after a heavy meal, before exercising. Make sure you drink plenty of fluid 10 to 15 minutes before you start (see "Drink Up" below). And don't forget the warm-up. This can consist of a few gentle repeats of head and shoulder circling, arm swinging, knee bending and ankle flexing. At the end of this, the pulse should be raised slightly. Don't stop suddenly after hard aerobics either, if you don't want to feel giddy. A few minutes of slowing down, walking gently perhaps on the spot, and a repeat of the warm-up are the ideal. A warm bath after vigorous exercising can soothe sore muscles.

DRINK UP

Thirst is not a good indicator of short-term body needs. We feel sufficiently refreshed before our true needs are met. This means a quenching drink after a hot workout will not be sufficient replenishment. Body perspiration is evaporated on the skin surface, and replacement through drinking fluids prevents dehydration, an early sign of which is fatigue. To replace fluids adequately, drink two large glasses of water (15 fluid oz) 10 to 15 minutes before you start a highly energetic workout, and one additional glass (6 to 8 fluid oz) every 15 to 20 minutes during exercise. Water is best, but if you prefer soft drinks or fruit juices, water them down, because the sugar content slows absorption.

CHECKING YOUR PULSE RATE

Before starting an aerobic sport or an aerobics program, find your safety level by checking your pulse. The aim of aerobic exercise is to raise the pulse rate by making the heart beat faster in order to strengthen the heart and increase stamina.

To gain this benefit, you have to maintain the higher rate for a specific length of time; however, doing too much too soon can be dangerous, causing heart strain, so the process of building up stamina will vary according to age and ability.

Press the artery on the outside of your wrist, below the thumb, using the tips of your third and fourth fingers. Or press on the carotid artery, which is in the side of the neck. Use a digital watch or a clock with a second hand to count the number of beats a minute. You might want to do this over a period of 30 seconds and double your finding. Or do it twice, making sure you are genuinely relaxed. What you will have is your resting heart rate.

The normal, healthy rate for the 50-to-60 age group is 67 or fewer beats per minute; for over 60 years it is 69 or fewer beats. Above 75 to 80 beats could mean stress or ill health, though injury or emotional upset can make the pulse rate temporarily extra high. Athletes and very fit people may have a slower pulse, around 50 beats per minute. A very slow pulse, 35 beats or fewer, can be associated with heart disease or other illness.

Now jog on the spot for one minute, stop, and immediately take your pulse again. This is your working heart rate.

To get the normal or average working heart rate for your age, take the figure of 220 beats per minute and simply subtract your age. So for a 45 year old, you get a maximum pulse rate of 175 beats per minute; for a 50 year old it will be 170; for a 60 year old 160, and so on.

When you calculate your own rate, it may not measure up to anything like this if you are unused to aerobic exercise. The aim, in any case, is not to reach the maximum "ideal" but to work within 60 percent to 80 percent of it. Some people find this too much, but even working to 50 percent will improve general fitness.

When first starting aerobics, try just 6 minutes of exercise at first, building up over two or three weeks to 15 minutes. You can check your pulse to monitor your progress.

Don't continue if you feel any intense strain—see the danger pointers in "Playing Safe—Recognizing and Avoiding Risks," later in this chapter.

TYPES OF AEROBIC ACTIVITY

You don't have to jog to get aerobic fitness. Here are three popular alternatives that will have the same effect, and more.

WALKING

All you need is reasonably dry weather and, ideally, a local hill or two. You can walk in the winter and summer. Wear light, layered clothing, so you can take something off if you get hot. A light windbreaker, with a hood, is better than a heavy coat. Shoes are best if they are waterproof—even in summer, the ground in some areas can be wet from rain or heavy dew. Tough hiking boots are only necessary for hill climbing in wintry conditions. Modern walking shoes are often lightweight and supple, but tennis shoes are sufficient for walking on paths and in parkland, as long as they have adequate cushioning, soles that grip and sides that give ankle support.

Walking is essentially do-it-yourself stuff, but some gyms are beginning to offer special instruction, either outdoors or using a treadmill. They may create a three-level program starting with walking at the rate of two miles an hour for perhaps 15 minutes, during which time novices are asked to check that their backs are straight, there is no hollowing below the waist, their shoulders are back and down, and their head and chest are up. This slow start is in effect the warm-up. Then comes the second level, walking at four miles an hour, which will induce aerobic activity in most people. Arm swinging and pumping is added. The third level is for the very fit, at five or more miles an hour, and various foot movements and hip rolling techniques are added. The Balboa system, founded in the Walking Center in New York, emphasizes leg straightening to full capacity when striding, with arms following leg movement.

If you are a self-starter, time yourself and gradually build up from two to three miles an hour until you can do two miles in 30 minutes, and then extend to an hour's walking. Always take the first 15 minutes slowly, for the warm-up. If you don't get aerobic breathlessness at four miles an hour, push yourself faster or find a more challenging route. Keep to a regular route for the first few weeks, so you can monitor your progress accurately.

Walking is about the safest exercise you can do, but you can feel strain from your feet pounding the ground instead of lifting off rhythmically, back arching or hunched shoulders. A swing in the stride, with arms to match, upright posture and relaxed shoulders take the strain away from the lower back.

EXERCISE IN BED WITH A MORNING STRETCH

Start flat on your back, stretch your legs down, arms out sideways. Bend your right leg up so the thigh is upright and the shin is parallel with the ceiling. Bring the bent knee down as far as possible over the left outstretched leg. Hold your knee down with your left hand and keep shoulders flat and back. Repeat with the other leg. Bring both knees up to your chest and hug them to you with your arms. Bend your knees so your feet are flat on the bed and lift off with buttocks. Turn your head slowly to the right, then the left. Spend a few seconds on each stretch, repeating two to three times.

TENNIS

This could take over from walking as the number-one option for the over-50s. Enthusiasts point out that you get training in aerobic work, agility, speedy responses and also mental alertness, which may generate connections between brain neurons to keep the mind young. There are even claims that the pattern of a typical game, with bursts of stress followed by recovery, is a useful preparation for the ups and downs of daily life.

Flexibility is necessary to prevent injury and to make for a smooth game, and today yoga-type stretches and body-twist exercises are part of the training for professionals. W. Ben Kibler, a member of the U.S. Tennis Association sports-science committee, recommends specific stretch areas: shoulder and elbow of the striking arm, hips and lower back. You also need flexibility in the Achilles tendon and calf muscles. Stretches should be part of the warm-up and, for a fast recovery, also the cool-down after playing.

DANCING

You can go to a dance class, buy a video for home use or try the following routine.

First, choose your music. Pick a slow, regular beat to start with—you can progress to a fast beat later. Stretch one arm and concentrate on stretching your hand and wrist as you move to the rhythm. Then bring the other arm into the picture, smoothly moving and stretching to your sides, in front and above your head. Now bring movement to the head, rolling gently to the music. Bend and sway from the waist, concentrating first on the upper body, then bringing in your hips. Keep your feet still on the floor and move and stretch with the rest of your body, including your legs. Finally let yourself go and move everything however you want.

PLAYING SAFE—
RECOGNIZING AND AVOIDING RISKS

Intense training of the international/competitive kind can weaken the immune system. Women athletes can become anorexic, lose bone density and stop having periods through overexercise. Some long-distance runners have dropped dead on the circuit. Even vigorous exercise at a nonprofessional level can be hazardous. A survey of men aged 40 to 59 who took part in physical activities showed that when it was moderate, such as frequent walking, it added no risk to those with or without a history of heart disease. However, when it was vigorous, there was an increased risk of heart attack in both groups. In midlife, only those who have exercised vigorously on a regular basis since their younger days are safe to keep up the pace.

For those who stick to the slower lanes, exercise is safe as long as you take reasonable precautions, which start with getting a doctor's go-ahead if there are any health doubts, such as rheumatoid disorders, severe osteoporosis, heart conditions or chronic infectious diseases. Exercise may be very much on the agenda with some of these medical conditions, but it might have to be of a certain kind, possibly under supervision.

Don't exercise when suffering from an acute infection. Coughs and sore throats are warning signs that the body needs resting, not challenging, as does a temperature of 99.5° F or over.

NO ACHING BONES

"I don't have an aching bone in my body," claimed Mrs. Elizabeth Huntley Flindt, at the age of 94. In younger days, she was a competition-winning modern ballroom dancer, gaining several top awards. Golf, daily exercise—"even when waiting for the teakettle to boil"— and of course dancing remained part of her life long after the prizes stopped. "I walk very fast, never stroll round the shops. I could probably still walk at four miles an hour."

Erratic participation in vigorous activity by sedentary individuals in the over-50 age group carries a high risk of heart problems, says the Carnegie Health Report. Trouble can occur when the exercise regime is too intense and when there is little warm-up or cool-down. Anyone doing vigorous exercise should know how to recognize the warning signs of heart problems. These symptoms may not point to a heart problem, but should be checked out. Watch out for the following:

- pain or discomfort in the chest
- feeling of nausea during or after exercising, sudden breathlessness at a level of exercise that normally seems easy
- dizziness and fainting while exercising (not when stopping, which can be due to insufficient cool-down), irregular pulse when pulse is normally regular
- very rapid heart rate when resting—say 100 beats per minute after five minutes of rest

Patients with coronary heart disease may well be prescribed exercise as part of their rehabilitation program. A great deal of evidence now shows the benefits both in terms of long-term mortality and general well-being. There are Heart Rate Monitor devices that can be programmed by physicians to individual needs and give warnings when an activity is creating too much strain.

Hyperthermia, overheating of the body during exercise, could lead to heatstroke, which is sometimes fatal. Signs to watch for are headache, dizziness, lack of balance, nausea, cramps, disorientation and excessive or irregular sweating. If the weather is hot and humid, outdoor exercise should be moderated. Drink extra fluid before, during and after exercising (see "Drink Up" on page 19).

If muscles feel sore and ache slightly after exercising, give yourself a rest for a day or two. The aches can sometimes start a couple of days after the exercise session, and continue for several days. When you resume exercising, take things a little more easily. As muscles adapt, aches and stiffness usually disappear.

Joint injury is a much more serious matter, and can lead to permanent damage to your spine, hips and knees. Jogging, racquetball and other fast competitive games as well as skipping can cause problems, often because of shoes that do not absorb the impact of pounding on hard surfaces. Running shoes should have high shock absorbency, stability and firm support. And even expensive models need replacing after covering about 500 miles.

Some people have one leg longer than the other or an uneven gait that makes them put too much weight on the inner or outer side of the foot. This "defect" may only show up in runners, who then experience joint problems. If in doubt, consult a sports-injury specialist or sports-shoe specialist. A safer alternative for joggers prone to injury and over-50s who want to avoid joint wear and tear is trampoline jumping, which retains the aerobic element but avoids the heavy impact on joints.

If you suffer a sudden injury, like a torn ligament or fracture, you may need to avoid stress on the area affected for just a day or two, or you may need to rest for several weeks, depending on the seriousness of the injury. Consult a doctor or sports-injury expert if the pain persists or gets worse after 48 hours of rest. Don't exercise again until any swelling has subsided and the injured area can take your weight or any pressure without increasing pain. Return slowly to exercising with stretching and possibly weight training first and a careful warm-up, then cut back on your old routine by half, gradually building up to your former exercise level in 10 percent increments.

CHAPTER TWO

The Nutrition Challenge

ARE YOU WHAT YOU EAT?

Gather together a selection of articles reflecting current thinking about healthy eating and you'll get a very mixed bunch of ideas: There's the fashionable Mediterranean diet—lots of fruit, vegetables and olive oil to guard against heart disease; you'll also find debate on the virtues of fiber, the importance of fish, the dangers of meat and the advantages of vegetarianism. And then we have the conflicting views on the value of a low-fat diet, the pros and cons of alcohol consumption, the controversy over vitamin supplements and antioxidants, the calcium needs of post-menopausal women and the arguments over proposed dietary restriction, based on the fact that rats on a low-calorie diet live longer.

Nutrition is a confusing area today, with many rules and theories competing for attention and validity. Although eating may seem like a fundamental simple pleasure, in fact it is a complex process. There are two sayings that sum up most of our attitudes about food. One is that "a little of what you crave does you good," which is liberal and associated with pleasure, and carries within it that modern moral, the *right* to eat what you like. It suggests that food is about choice, social interaction and escape from rules and theories.

The other, "you are what you eat," is darker, and moral in a more traditional sense. It is saying you are good if you eat good food, bad if you don't, and threatens you with the consequences if you make the wrong choice. If you choose bad food, you get the health you deserve. Most of us would prefer to resist this spoilsport approach. We'd like to think, without thinking too hard, that we eat a balanced, healthy diet without bothering too much about the rules. We may resent the interference of experts who want to change our eating habits, and who can't even make up their own minds about what is good and bad.

DO WE NEED TO WORRY ABOUT VITAMINS AND MINERALS?

Governments in many countries set desired levels of vitamins and minerals. Daily intake below these levels is thought to expose people to malnutrition and disease. However, these levels, though revised from time to time, differ in different countries. The Recommended Daily Allowances (RDA) in the United States, for instance, tend to be higher than the Dietary Reference Values (DRV) in the United Kingdom. (For a complete table of U.S. recommendations, see "Vitamins and Minerals— The Complete List" at the end of this chapter.) Gerontologists—scientists who study the aging process and the old as a social group—are beginning to question whether current recommended allowances are relevant to older people, since we become less efficient at metabolizing vitamins as we age. Evidence also points to differing needs in different circumstances. We absorb more vitamins when our needs are greater— extra vitamin C, for instance, may be utilized when we have a cold (it is now understood to relieve symptoms rather than prevent colds). Smokers, heavy drinkers and women taking oral contraceptives metabolize vitamin C less efficiently than do others, and therefore need higher amounts to compensate. The question as to whether women on HRT, or others on long-term medication, also need higher amounts has not been explored. These facts are making some nutrition experts revise their views that people in Western countries are, if anything, over- rather than undernourished.

> *"The only advice I can give about having a long life is to get a good, mixed diet and a job you like."*
>
> —*Susie Cooper, pottery designer, aged 90*

In fact, there is evidence that older people don't get all the nutrients they need. The Baltimore Longitudinal Study on Aging found deficiencies among elderly people in calcium, zinc, iron, magnesium, vitamins B_6, B_{12}, D and E, and in folic acid. A survey from England revealed that pressure sores in elderly patients with thigh fractures were associated with low blood levels of vitamin C. (As many as 60 percent of patients with such fractures develop pressure sores, and there's some evidence that vitamin C supplements improve healing.)

How careless—or carefree—can we afford to be about our daily diet? It would be foolish to ignore modern advice on "good" and "bad" foods on the basis that our foremothers and forefathers managed without it. They also managed without the degree of pollution, pesticides and food additives that we are exposed to. But they were sometimes victims of ignorance. Lack of vitamin D produced rickets; lead from glazing in cooking pots leached into food to cause toxic effects; beef and pork were sometimes infested with tapeworm before standards of hygiene were introduced; lack of vitamin C resulted in scurvy. Eating by instinct is not necessarily good for you.

Perhaps the answer is tailor-made diets, ones that would reflect our individual nutritional needs according to age, sex, body chemistry and genetic strengths and weaknesses. Maybe that's what we'll get one day. For the time being, we can only pick and choose by being informed.

The rest of the chapter examines in detail current ideas about eating and offers practical advice. If you find yourself irritated, confused or even downright hostile, stick with it. This is important reading for your future health. Once you know the available information, you can recognize the vulnerable areas in your eating pattern and make your choices and compromises. In "Summing up—Guidelines for the Best Possible Diet," at the end of the chapter, there is a list on all the points that have been covered. After that it's up to you.

EAT LESS, LIVE LONGER?

The big debate today among nutrition researchers is whether a low-calorie diet is the way to retard the aging process. The evidence goes back to the 1930s when Clive McCay and his colleagues restricted the food intake of young rats and found that those who survived the first year lived much longer than rats that were allowed to eat as much as they liked. The current revival of interest in dietary restriction supports those early findings and suggests that changes associated with aging and age-linked diseases are slowed down by eating a low-calorie diet, the result being an increase in lifespan of up to 50 percent.

Of course, we're talking about rats, mice and, more recently, fruit flies, but not too many humans. It's not easy to monitor humans over a life span on a restricted diet. The people of Okinawa, Japan, provide one of the few pieces of evidence on the advantages of dietary restriction. For cultural, and possibly economic, reasons they have existed on a diet consisting largely of fish and green vegetables, with a total calorie content at least 20 percent lower than the rest of Japan. They suffer significantly lower rates of cancer, heart disease and stroke than their compatriots and their average life span is increased in that they have a higher proportion of centenarians. However, their maximum possible life span is no greater than anywhere else, and critics of the dietary-restriction theory point out that fish and green vegetables offer protection against heart disease and cancer in any case, and a low-calorie diet in and of itself may not be beneficial.

Current clinical work is getting nearer to humans, focusing on primates in the form of rhesus and squirrel monkeys. At the National Institute of Health Animal Center in Maryland, there are two groups of monkeys growing up on two different diets, one consisting of 30 percent fewer calories than the other. At about the age of six, maturation (in the form of skeletal development and the onset of puberty) was delayed by about 18 months in the dieting monkeys. As the monkeys age, scientists will be examining everything from cell changes to fingernail growth. We can expect to learn a lot more about the anti-aging mechanisms of dietary restriction in the next few years.

EIGHT MEALS A DAY: IT'S OKAY

Eating little and often may be healthier than eating three meals a day, as long as the snacking is health-conscious. Frequent small meals can benefit the heart by significantly reducing cholesterol levels—the only catch is that the snacks have to number eight or more a day. The advantage of this way of eating lies in the fact that nutrients enter the body at a slower rate and therefore the process may be less demanding than if you were eating three full meals daily.

Meanwhile, the evidence for dietary restriction is certainly impressive as far as rats and mice are concerned, with the development of all diseases and tumors prevented or slowed down during their longer life span. These effects may not be due to the decrease of body fat or protein, or to the reduction of the metabolic rate. The current view is that the crucial factor is simply reducing calorie intake. This may influence either the endocrine (hormonal) system or the nervous system, changing the way the calories are used as energy by the body.

Could we, or should we, start cutting calories now, before all the evidence is in? Dietary restriction, so long as it is nutritionally sound, has no adverse effects on humans. Researchers in this field say there is no reason why the consistently positive results in other mammals should not also occur in humans, even when the diet is started in later life.

HOW MUCH DO WE NEED?

A reasonable interpretation of dietary restriction for humans is between 1500 and 2000 calories daily. Roy Walford of the University of California at Los Angeles, one of the enthusiasts in this field, put himself on a diet of 1600 calories in 1984 when he was around the age of 60. Now, according to press reports, his intake has gone up to 2100 calories daily.

A life on low calories may be longer lasting, but it's not much fun. A compromise would be to cut back to between 1500 and 2000 calories for several weeks now and then. Variations must depend on body build and amount of energy consumed in daily life. Perhaps more important is the quality, rather than quantity, of calories. What should constitute the calories you eat is the subject of the rest of the chapter.

FREE RADICALS & ANTIOXIDANTS—WHY YOU NEED TO KNOW ABOUT THEM

The free radical theory of aging holds that certain molecules are responsible for the bodily changes that occur as we age. These molecules, the most common of which are oxygen-free radicals, are produced by cells in the body. Free radicals are by-products of normal metabolism, made when cells turn food and oxygen into energy, and they set up a damaging chain reaction that changes a cell's shape or function. They are not all bad, and in small amounts may even help the immune system, but some researchers believe that they cause tissues and organs to age, and may also trigger degenerative disorders including cancer, hardening of the arteries, cataracts and Alzheimer's disease.

Antioxidants are substances that react with the oxygen-free radicals and disarm them. We get antioxidants from a number of sources, including vitamins C and E and beta-carotene, and from enzymes (proteins produced by the body). Antioxidants can prevent much of the damage caused by free radicals, which is why we should include plenty of them in our diet.

There is also an enzyme called SOD (superoxide dismutase), which appears to convert free radicals into the also harmful hydrogen peroxide, which is then made harmless by another enzyme. SOD, then, is a good thing. Research on fruit flies has shown that if you insert extra copies of the SOD gene into them, they will live 5 to 10 percent longer than average. At the National Institute on Aging, scientist Richard Cutler has found that SOD levels are directly related to life span in 20 different species. Longer-living animals have higher levels of SOD, which leads to the idea that the ability to fight free radicals is linked to longer life spans. Though not yet proven, this theory looks promising.

A compound called PBN, which works in ways similar to beta-carotene, has been found to slow down the aging process in gerbils. Researchers Robert A. Floyd at the Oklahoma Medical Research Foundation and John H. Carney at the University of Kentucky gave PBN to young adult and older gerbils and found that, after two weeks, the levels of free radicals in the older group were reduced to levels comparable with the younger animals. The younger group did not benefit, and once the treatment ended, the levels of free radicals gradually rose again in the older animals.

EATING RIGHT: A GOOD EXAMPLE

Topol, the actor, always carries a supply of dried fruit, whole-grain bread and mineral water in case he gets hungry. In his 60s, he still takes on the grueling role of Tevye in *Fiddler on the Roof*, keeping fit by running several miles every day and eating large amounts of fresh fruits, raw vegetables and salads. "I never eat red meat and no oil, but I hate to preach," he says. His favorite drinks are water and apple juice, and an occasional beer or glass of wine.

For the present, these findings hold only slim promises for humans. SOD taken in tablet form is simply broken down in the human digestive system. Perhaps one day PBN will turn out to be a safe and effective supplement, but it is still too early to say. And antioxidant vitamins, when added to cells, leave free radicals unchanged.

Even so, there are signs that vitamins do work as antioxidants. Vitamin C is thought to protect against heart disease by blocking oxidation of cholesterol-carrying proteins and thus reducing the chances of arteriosclerosis (hardening of the arteries). Vitamin E may protect arteries in a similar way, and adequate daily amounts of both are accepted by the medical profession as important in the fight against heart disease.

Does this mean we should be taking vitamin supplements, or merely ensuring a high vitamin intake in our daily diet? The answers are by no means straightforward, as the next section illustrates.

VITAMINS AGAINST AGING— NO DOUBT ABOUT IT

The vitamin supplement market is booming, particularly among 45 to 64 year olds. In the United States we're talking of a market of 100 million people. This may be good news for vitamin manufacturers, but doctors, on the whole, don't like it. Why vitamins, they say, when we can get the nutrients in our normal diet? Why megadoses, when there is no substantial proof that they do any good and some proof that they can be dangerous? Despite the proliferation of theories and findings on the benefits of vitamin supplements, the medical profession holds back. (One exception that most doctors agree on is that pregnant women cannot get sufficient folic acid in a normal diet and need it in supplement form to protect against neural tube defects in pregnancy.) Vitamin popping may be popular with the public, but it's out in the cold as far as most of the medical profession is concerned.

Yet research repeatedly points to the benefits of vitamins A, C, E and beta-carotene supplements in protecting against heart disease, cancer and cataracts. Around 3000 research studies have been compiled by the Bristol Cancer Help Center database, all of them the work of "prestigious scientists and laboratories, published in mainstream medical journals," according to Sandra Goodman, the compiler. Here are a few findings:

- Vitamin E, beta-carotene and the mineral selenium, taken as supplements, reduced by 13 percent the number of expected deaths from cancer in a five-year study of 30,000 Chinese. Several groups were involved, one taking the vitamin E in combination as above, another taking vitamin A and zinc, a third taking the B vitamins with riboflavin and niacin, and a fourth taking vitamin C and yeast. Only in the vitamin E group did cancer rates drop significantly. But in the vitamin B group there was a 41 percent reduction in cataracts. (The province of Linxian, where the study took place, has very high rates of stomach and esophageal cancer, and is an area where fruit and vegetables are in short supply.)

- Taking vitamin E supplements of 100 or more international units (IU) a day cut the risk of heart disease in a large group of female nurses by 46 percent, according to Dr. Meir Stampfer of the Harvard School of Public Health. The 87,000-strong study was conducted over a period of two years and showed that those taking vitamin E were half as likely to develop heart disease as the nontakers. Another Harvard study showed that vitamin E reduced the incidence of expected heart attacks by 50 percent in 333 male physicians with known heart disease.

- In a review of 156 studies published in the medical journal *Nutrition and Cancer*, lack of fruit and vegetable consumption was clearly associated with cancer risk. The protective effect of fruits and vegetables helped prevent lung, pancreatic, stomach, bowel, cervical and breast cancer. Fruits and vegetables contain antioxidant vitamins C and E, beta-carotenes, folic acid, fiber, selenium and other micronutrients. Vitamin C is thought to limit stomach cancer by reducing nitrites in water and food.

- Low blood levels of vitamin E and beta-carotene are associated with increased risk of breast, cervical and lung cancer in a variety of trials carried out in the United States and England. Supplements of vitamins A, C and E were found to improve the auto-immune system in 30 elderly hospitalized patients. A matched group given placebo or dummy supplements showed no similar benefits. Similar findings come from a study of 96 elderly couples living independently. After a year on multivitamin supplements, they had improved immunity and less infection than a placebo-treated group. A boost to the immune system can reduce infection-related illness by 50 percent.

- Cataracts are less likely to develop in people aged 40 and over if they take antioxidant vitamins E and C, plus beta-carotene. In one study by researchers Edwin Bunce and John Hess of the State University of Blacksburg, Virginia, a group with cataracts was matched with a cataract-free group, and the latter was found to take significantly more vitamins C and E. There was a 70 percent decrease in cataract risk in subjects taking vitamin C supplements compared to nontakers, and a 56 percent decrease in cataract risk in those taking vitamin E supplements compared to nontakers.

- Exercise can increase free radicals. The evidence comes from observation of exercise-exhausted animals who had raised levels of free radicals in the liver and in muscles, including the heart. Several studies of exercising humans show that damage attributed to increased free radical activity can be prevented by taking vitamin E supplements.

- Antioxidant levels are depleted by up to 30 percent in the blood of smokers as compared to nonsmokers. This may be partly due to poor eating habits, but it is also attributed to the negative effect of smoking itself. Unfortunately, a survey published in the *New England Journal of Medicine* reported that 29,000 smokers taking supplements of vitamin E and beta-carotene showed no decrease in cancer or heart disease other than a significant reduction of prostate cancer. The authors of the report suggest that vegetables may contain other, as yet unidentified, ingredients that the supplement they monitored may not contain. Other commentators reflect that damage from a lifetime of smoking cannot be reversed that easily.

SHOULD WE BE TAKING
VITAMIN SUPPLEMENTS?

Until recently, vitamin supplements were thought to be strictly for health nuts. The orthodox opinion was that almost everyone gets enough vitamins in a normal diet. Now, with the antioxidant effect taken seriously, no one is really sure. There is still too much theory resting on too little knowledge. Research is in progress in a big way, but for the present we have no more to go on than a few guidelines and a lot of opinions.

There is no doubt that research into diet is expanding. The American National Institute on Aging is continuing to sponsor work on antioxidants. British cancer-research charities are examining the British diet and comparing it to that of other European countries while also comparing mortality rates. Oxford University, with the British Heart Foundation, is also investigating antioxidant vitamins and looking at intake of orange juice in childhood and its effect on coronary arteries in later life. There are many new initiatives that aim to increase our understanding of the effects of vitamins.

FOR SUPPLEMENTS . . .

Here is a selection of quotes from respected scientists who have publicly supported vitamin supplements:

"I advocate antioxidant vitamin and zinc supplements in treatment of age-related macular degeneration (i.e., cataract) because it may be helpful and poses minimal risk."—*Dr. David Newsome, Tulane University* (Medical World News, *January 1993*).

"There's ample evidence that nutrients can help [prevent cancer and other diseases]. . . . It is a public health mistake to limit our efforts to fruits and vegetables and tell people not to take supplements."—*Gladys Block, Professor of Public Health Nutrition, University of California (Report from 4th International Congress on Anti-Carcinogenesis and Radiation Protection at Johns Hopkins University, Baltimore, 18–23 April 1993).*

"Supplementing the diet may be sensible for children and for people who lead busy lives."—*Dr. Catherine Rice-Evans, Guy's and St. Thomas' Medical School, London (*The Independent, *15 September 1993).*

"I think we have enough data in hand for physicians to begin suggesting their patients take supplements, or at least not discourage them from it."—*Jeffrey Blumberg, Professor of Nutrition and Associate Director of USDA's Human Nutrition Research Center on Aging, Tufts University* (Medical World News, *January 1993).*

"Although the data is incomplete, it is possible to put forward values for intake of [those] nutrients that would be expected to provide the lowest risk of disease . . . we should encourage rather than discourage people to take a modest natural supplement."—*Anthony Diplock, Professor of Biochemistry at the University of London at Guy's Hospital ("Antioxidant Nutrients as Preventive Agents in Human Disease: A Position of Statement," June 1992).*

. . . AND AGAINST

Notes of caution are struck by other, equally respected scientists, the main objection to vitamins being that the evidence is not totally convincing and considerably more research is needed before specific dietary advice should be given to the general public. Critics also point out that the high doses of vitamins needed to achieve the protective effects found in most of the trials put them into a category far exceeding a natural supplement. The vitamins reach the status of a drug, and might have a toxic effect if taken regularly.

This is particularly true of those vitamins that are stored in the body. In high doses, vitamin A can cause liver damage, joint pains, blurred vision and headaches, risks to be balanced against the discovery that it can also promote normal cell growth and help prevent lung cancer. (Useful for smokers, though nothing is as effective as stopping smoking.) Massive doses of B_6, taken for premenstrual tension, can cause dizziness and neurological damage. Vitamin B_{12}, taken to cure pernicious anemia, is stored in the liver and would be toxic in anything but small amounts. Vitamin D is stored in the body, not passed in urine if unused, so large amounts can accumulate in tissues and have a toxic effect. Too much vitamin D can also cause kidney stones.

In contrast, the antioxidant vitamins C, E and beta-carotene are not stored. Surplus amounts are passed in the urine. However, a regular intake of several grams of vitamin C daily could, in rare cases, cause kidney stones in people already susceptible. High levels of vitamin C also stimulate iron absorption, which is good for most people, but not for a few individuals suffering from a faulty iron-storing condition.

And abruptly stopping megadoses of vitamin C can cause temporary withdrawal resulting in scurvy-type symptoms. Vitamin E in high doses does not appear to cause problems, and the only known side effect of beta-carotene is that in very large amounts it can turn the skin a yellowish shade, most noticeable on the palms and soles of feet. This, however, is harmless.

WHICH SUPPLEMENTS TO CHOOSE

Judging by the research so far, the protective effects of antioxidant vitamins are derived from daily intake of at least 100 international units (IUs) of vitamin E and 300 mg of vitamin C—far more than we can get in our normal diet, and therefore more than any recommended daily allowances set by governments. For those not taking part in research trials, there are few guidelines. Jeffrey Blumberg, quoted above, advocates a "broad-based multivitamin, multimineral supplement formulated at one or two times the RDA . . . a conservative and rational thing to do for older people." Linus Pauling, a two-time Nobel prize winner and champion of vitamin C who lived to the age of 93, took 18,000 milligrams of vitamin C per day for several years, and also 800 IU of vitamin E, plus extra B vitamins, beta-carotene and vitamin A.

ANTIOXIDANT VITAMINS

These figures for ideal daily intake are for adults. Amounts may differ for children, and for pregnant and lactating women.

Recommended Daily Allowances

Vitamin A as beta-carotene	2666–3333 IU
Retinal equivalent	800–1000 mcg
Vitamin C	60 mg
Vitamin E	8–10 mcg

Striking a more moderate note, Dr. Catherine Rice-Evans suggests that if you want to take daily supplements, select from brands that give 75 mg of vitamin E (the equivalent of around 115 IU), 100 mg of vitamin C and 15 mg of beta-carotene. And Professor Anthony Diplock suggests 50 to 80 mg of vitamin E (the equivalent of 75 to 120 IU), 100 to 150 mg of vitamin C and 15 to 25 mg of beta-carotene.

THE BEST ONES TO BUY

What you see is definitely not what you get from a vitamin supplement. Whatever the dose stated on the pack, only a small proportion of the potency is actually absorbed. Far more disconcerting is the discovery that many vitamin supplements on the market are virtually useless because they fail to dissolve in the stomach and are excreted. Two surveys conducted in England and published in the British *Food Magazine* showed that vitamins and minerals that take longer than 20 minutes to dissolve remain in large granules in the stomach where they stay, without releasing their good effects, until excreted. A survey from the Washington-based Center for Science in the Public Interest showed similar findings.

The vitamin supplement buyer needs to look on the package for words like "rapidly digested" or "fast dissolving," or, where possible, to choose chewable supplements. Multivitamins in line with full RDA vitamins, minerals and trace elements are sometimes prescribed by doctors (usually for those found to be nutritionally deficient) and are also available over the counter.

In the not-too-distant future, we may be buying supplements in a totally new way. Scientists are predicting the development of a new range of "fortified" foods. They will resemble their distant cousins, the fortified breads and breakfast cereals, and vitamin-enriched fruit juices, etc., but are likely to have higher amounts of nutrients, in line with the current theories on disease prevention. Already, fiber-enriched drinks, calcium-added chewing gum, and salad dressings with anticholesterol additions are popular in Japan. Folic acid may soon be recommended for all women of child-bearing age, and might be added to a staple food such as bread.

ANTIOXIDANTS FROM NATURAL SOURCES

Most people in developed countries eat foods containing antioxidants on a regular basis, but not in very large quantities. Though the protective results come mainly from supplements in amounts larger than what we normally eat, there is some evidence to show that increasing our intake of fruits and vegetables will also do the trick. A study of over 400 cases of rectal cancer showed the protective effect of carotene, vitamin C and dietary fiber from vegetables (not cereals). Cancer risk decreased with raised intakes of broccoli, carrots, celery, cucumber, green peppers, lettuce and tomatoes.

Vitamin C comes from fresh fruit and vegetables, especially dark green and red ones, and citrus fruits. Root vegetables contain good amounts of vitamin C, but there are seasonal variations. New potatoes, for instance, can contain up to three times as much as older ones that are stored and eaten in winter. Vitamin C is easily lost through storage, cooking and even the cutting of potatoes. If you leave potatoes to soak in water before boiling, or overcook cabbage, you can lose up to 75 percent of the vitamin. Vegetables kept hot for half an hour or more after cooking lose even more. Freezing, however, has no depleting effect. Dried fruits contain little or no vitamin C.

Vitamin E is present in vegetable oils, such as safflower and soybean oil, in nuts and in whole-grain wheat, rice and oats. Heating and storing does not have a negative effect, but food processing that removes the bran reduces the nutrient value and is the reason why whole-grain breads are considered more nutritional than white bread.

Carotenes, the most potent of which are the beta-carotenes, occur naturally in foods and convert into vitamin A in the body. They are found chiefly in yellow and orange foods like carrots, sweet potatoes, apricots, pumpkin, cantaloupe melon, red and yellow peppers and also in dark green leafy vegetables such as spinach, watercress and fresh herbs. Carrot juice is an excellent source. Tomatoes contain beta-carotene, as well as an antioxidant called lycopene that is thought to enhance the absorption of beta-carotene. Beta-carotenes are not normally lost in cooking. (Vitamin A is also converted from retinol, derived from liver, egg yolk, fish liver oil, butter and cheese. Margarines and other nonbutter fats are often fortified with vitamins A and D.)

How much of these foods should we be eating daily? The U.S. Department of Agriculture recommends 3 to 5 servings of vegetables, and 2 to 4 servings of fruit.

The emphasis here has been on the antioxidant vitamins. A balanced diet must include a variety of vitamins and minerals that interact with each other to enhance absorption. Some of these will be examined in detail, along with guidelines on the best eating for successful aging.

MINERALS FOR MENOPAUSE

Loss of bone begins in adulthood (from about the age of 35 in women) and accelerates at menopause, when a condition called osteoporosis may develop. Bone loss increases in the first five years after menopause, and then slows to a steady loss. Around 25 percent of women suffer this to a serious degree. The thinning of bone may eventually cause hip, spine, forearm or wrist fractures, and in elderly women can lead to infirmity and immense pain. Men lose bone as they age, too, but at a slower rate.

Calcium is a mineral that helps give bones their strength and rigidity. Almost all the calcium in our bodies is stored in bones. We need constant supplies of it to replace old bone and make new bone healthy. One possible reason for the high, and recently rising, incidence of osteoporosis is that we don't get enough calcium throughout life, so bone density is either already depleted at menopause or bone loss accelerates extra quickly at this time.

The combination of estrogen and calcium ensures bone strength, and loss normally remains gradual as long as the ovaries produce regular amounts of estrogen and the diet contains adequate amounts of calcium. But estrogen production from the ovaries ceases at menopause, and older people absorb vitamins and minerals less efficiently, so the amount of calcium metabolized is reduced.

Some doctors say that when there is no estrogen from the ovaries, taking extra calcium in the diet or in supplements is of little use. Only when hormone replacement therapy (HRT) is taken to restore premenopausal estrogen levels will the extra calcium be beneficial. (See "Menopause and After" in Chapter Three for more on HRT.)

A body of research contradicts this conclusion, and researchers are beginning to promote the idea of a calcium-rich diet after menopause as well as before it, not least because estrogen is still stored at low levels in the adrenal glands.

One trial reported in the *New England Journal of Medicine* covered 301 postmenopausal women, half on a usual dietary calcium intake of 400 to 650 mg a day, the others on less than 400 mg a day. Women in both groups were subdivided and given either a placebo or an extra 500 mg of calcium, using a form called calcium citrate. After two years, all of those women who had undergone menopause within the previous five years had lost bone from the spine, but not from thigh or forearm, whether they had been taking supplements or not. Those on calcium citrate, and longer past the menopause, experienced no significant bone loss in the period surveyed. A different subgroup taking calcium carbonate, another form of supplement, still lost bone from the spine but not from the other two sites. All the women who were further past menopause and had low dietary calcium intake experienced significantly greater bone loss.

There is some evidence that women who exercise and also get extra calcium in their diet maintain or gain bone density, even in old age. A screening and counseling project in New York followed up 53 women who were one to ten years past menopause. None were on HRT, all received at least 750 mg of calcium a day and undertook at least three hours of weight-bearing exercise a week. After a year to 18 months, bone density actually rose slightly in spine and thigh.

HOW MUCH CALCIUM?

Opinions differ about how much calcium postmenopausal women need, and a combination with vitamin D and magnesium may be as important as raising levels of calcium alone (see "The Case for Calcium Supplements" in this chapter). The recommended daily allowances of calcium differ for different age groups. The RDA ranges from 800 to 1200 mg daily for adults. An intake of over 2000 mg could create a dangerous nutritional imbalance.

CALCIUM-RICH FOODS

Milk, cheese and dairy products are the best sources of calcium, along with oily and canned fish, dark green vegetables, nuts, sesame seeds and dried fruit. There is very little calcium in meat and not much in lentils or similar dried legumes. Hard water contains calcium. Low-fat foods are as good a source as full-fat ones, if not better (see skimmed milk below). Here are some common foods with their calcium content (in milligrams):

300 ml (half pint) of whole milk	340 mg
300 ml (half pint) of skimmed milk	360 mg
small container of low-fat yogurt	225 mg
100 g (4 oz) cooked spinach	*170 mg
50 g (2 oz) sardines	220 mg
100 g (4 oz) canned salmon	106 mg
50 g (2 oz) cheddar cheese	415 mg
50 g (2 oz) cottage cheese	40 mg
100 g (4 oz) ice cream	134 mg
50 g (2 oz) chocolate	123 mg
1 large slice bread, white or whole-grain fortified	60 mg
100 g (4 oz) broccoli, boiled	46 mg
50 g (2 oz) dried apricots	52 mg
1 medium size egg	40 mg
50 g (2 oz) lentils, cooked	9 mg
l large orange	58 mg
50 g (2 oz) peanuts	34 mg
50 g (2 oz) almonds	125 mg
25 g (1 oz) sesame seed	190 mg

* Absorption of calcium is impaired in some foods, especially vegetables, so although spinach is a useful source, it is not as good as dairy products, despite its seemingly high calcium content.

You can get 1200 to 1500 mg of calcium from a daily diet as follows:

- at least 400 ml (two-thirds of a pint) of milk—take some of it in your morning cereal, also in coffee
- a cup of yogurt or 25 g (1 oz) cheddar cheese
- 4 slices of bread
- 2 helpings of dark green vegetables
- 2 pieces of fruit

This adds up to over 1000 mg, and the rest can come from fish, nuts, dried fruit, eggs, etc. You can get extra calcium by adding grated cheese to dishes, or yogurt to soups. Eat the bones in canned fish, such as sardines, to get the full calcium content.

THE CASE FOR CALCIUM SUPPLEMENTS

Extra calcium in the form of supplements seems to help the elderly more than those losing bone around the time of menopause. There's a body of evidence showing that women in their 70s and older can even regain bone by taking extra calcium, but there's nothing that's quite as encouraging for the first ten postmenopausal years. One study demonstrated that calcium supplementation significantly reduced bone loss in middle-aged women, particularly in the upper arm, but the research findings are not consistent.

Even so, if you're not sure you can get sufficient calcium from ordinary foods, it would make sense to consider a supplement at any time after menopause. Take it combined with vitamin D for optimum absorption. The combination of vitamin D and calcium has reduced fractures and increased bone density in women aged 70 and over. A trial involving more than 3000 women living in nursing homes or other care facilities resulted in 43 percent fewer hip fractures and 32 percent fewer wrist or forearm fractures in those given supplements compared to those given placebos. The supplements were 1 to 2 g of calcium and 800 IU of vitamin D for 18 months, and those taking them also had a 2.7 percent increase in thigh bone density while the untreated group had a 4.6 percent decrease.

With age, we become less efficient at utilizing vitamin D, and a deficiency may increase muscle weakness and contribute to falls and fractures. Also, some drugs interfere with vitamin absorption. If you take any drug regularly, ask your doctor about its effect.

When buying a supplement, check the label to be sure that you'll be taking at least 500 mg of calcium a day since the amount made available to the body is not the same as the actual dose stated on the package. The rest of the calcium needed should be made up through the diet. To complement the calcium, vitamin D intake should be around 400 IU. (The RDA for vitamin D is 200 to 400 IU.) There are different forms of calcium supplements. Calcium citrate is thought to be absorbed better than calcium carbonate, and chewable types are likely to be absorbed the most speedily.

The main dietary sources of vitamin D are oily fish such as herring, sardine and mackerel, and egg yolk, milk, butter and cod liver oil. Some foods such as breakfast cereals, margarines and skimmed milk powder are fortified with vitamin D—if so, the information will be on the package. We also get vitamin D from sunlight—you need exposure to the sun for half an hour a day, which is not considered a skin-cancer risk as long as sunscreen is used.

Remember that supplements for bones work best along with the bone-boosting effect of physical activity. See Chapter One for more information on exercise.

MAGNESIUM TOO?

If you take calcium and vitamin D, then you also need magnesium, claims Dr. Guy Abraham of the University of California, Los Angeles. He found that a supplement of 500 mg of calcium citrate and 600 mg of magnesium had a significant effect on reversing postmenopausal bone loss in women who were also taking HRT. The HRT-only takers experienced a 0.7-percent increase in bone density after 6 to 12 months of treatment, compared to an 11-percent increase on the combined regime. Dr. Abraham reasons that a chronic magnesium deficiency along with estrogen reduction is the cause of postmenopausal bone loss, and recommends daily calcium and magnesium, in amounts as above, plus 400 IU of vitamin D, from soon after menopause.

Dr. Abraham says the extra magnesium helps stabilize hormones that control calcium balance and increases the efficiency of vitamin D. Western diets, he claims, contain variable amounts of magnesium.

It must be said that most of the medical profession does not hold with the idea that we may be magnesium deficient, except in very rare cases. We get magnesium in the diet from potatoes, cabbage and other green vegetables, cheese, bread (whole-grain much more than white), bran, nuts, chocolate and dried fruit. And it also comes via the tap in drinking water, more in hard than in soft water, and in many bottled mineral waters.

What is generally accepted is that magnesium is necessary to absorb calcium properly. Recommended daily amounts range from 270 to 350 mg (much lower than the amount in Dr. Abraham's trial). Here are some magnesium-rich foods:

small bag of 24 cashew nuts	106 mg
small bag of 24 peanuts	45 mg
large slice of whole-grain bread	37 mg
handful of raisins	6 mg
2 medium boiled potatoes	30 mg
100 g (4 oz) roast chicken	28 mg
1 serving cauliflower	7 mg

If you choose to boost your intake of magnesium with a supplement, you'll find some included in multivitamin supplements that also contain antioxidants and calcium. Or you might look for a calcium/vitamin D/magnesium supplement.

BORON AND SILICON—THE HELPFUL TRACE ELEMENTS

If you think the decision-making process on supplements ends here, you are wrong. There are more minerals to explore.

A trace element called boron may help the body retain calcium. There have been some small studies suggesting that it reduces calcium and magnesium loss and increases estrogen levels if taken as a supplement, though the numbers of women involved in trials were very small. Boron exists in fruits such as apples and pears, as well as leafy vegetables and nuts, and is available in pill form at health food shops. There is no recommended daily level, though 3 mg is quoted by Maryon Stewart of the Women's Nutritional Advisory Service.

Another trace element, silicon, is said to "empower" calcium and therefore prevent osteoporosis, as well as strengthen nails and hair. There is no recommended daily requirement, but health writer Leslie Kenton claims we need as much as 20 to 30 mg, and though it is widespread in the soil we don't get enough of it. High-tech farming and modern food-processing are the culprits. Brown rice, whole-grain flour, fresh fruit eaten with the peel intact and organically grown products can provide silicon.

No single food or supplement or type of nutrient provides protection against osteoporosis. A healthy, balanced diet must include a variety of vitamins and minerals that interact for optimum absorption of calcium.

Some of the vitamins in the B group, such as folic acid, B_6 and B_{12}, are in poor supply in people with osteoporosis, says naturopath Leon Chaitow. He suspects that these vitamins may be involved with enzyme processes that influence the condition. Carbonated drinks and a diet high in red meats may supply too much phosphorus, which interferes with calcium absorption. However, there is some evidence that lower-income groups don't get sufficient phosphorous in the diet. Unprocessed bran may also reduce the effect of calcium.

High fluoride intake through drinking water is associated with a lower fracture rate and higher bone density. But a form of fluoride has been used as a treatment for osteoporosis without success in reducing fractures, and there is no reason to think that adding fluoride to the diet would be useful.

MINERALS FOR EVERYONE

If you believed everything you read from the fringe practitioners about the allegedly missing minerals in the average diet, you could easily conclude that you were seriously undernourished. As with vitamins, however, there's also the other school of thought—that a balanced diet gives us all the minerals we need. Who should we believe? It is not easy to find a middle ground between often under researched or over-optimistic claims on the one hand and steadfast conservatism on the other, but there are certain facts worth knowing. For instance:

- It is now scientifically acknowledged that long-term use of steroids interferes with calcium absorption, and this is distinct from the effect of the drop in estrogen after menopause.

- Nonsteroidal anti-inflammatory drugs, often taken by the elderly for arthritis, may require a higher-than-normal iron intake in order to prevent anemia.

- Iron deficiency in women during heavy periods and after childbirth is well known, as is zinc deficiency in the Western diet.

- One survey showed that low-income families had low intakes of calcium, phosphorus and magnesium, to which women in the same economic group could add potassium, iodine and zinc.

- Selenium, a mineral trace element that enhances antioxidants, is thought to be plentiful in Western diets since it is present in the soil, yet northern European agricultural land is among the poorest in selenium in the world, and in Finland selenium is added to artificial fertilizers in recognition of this.

IMPORTANT MINERALS

Here's a closer look at some of the minerals that are claimed to be missing from our lives. Some are widely available in everyday foods, so if you have a balanced diet the conservatives are likely to be right in their assertion that you don't need a supplement. But other minerals occur only in less common foods and a borderline deficiency is not out of the question. If you want to play it safe by taking a multivitamin and mineral supplement, check the ingredients on the label. Recommended daily allowances are given at the end of the chapter. Minerals complement each other in complex ways and a high intake of any single mineral could be toxic.

GINSENG—NATURALLY ANTI-AGING

Doctors in the West don't take ginseng seriously. But they do in Russia, where it has been used to boost stamina after finding soldiers who took it did better in athletic performance than those given a placebo. Ginseng root is known to contain a stimulant that can alleviate fatigue and may help to combat stress. Whether it also promotes longevity is open to debate. It can be taken as a booster for a month once or twice a year—no longer than that since it may raise blood pressure and cause insomnia. Siberian ginseng is considered the best, followed by Korean and Chinese, and then Japanese. Roots, root pieces and extracts are far more potent than tablets, powders and teas.

Iodine is not plentiful in our diet. We can get it from fish and seafoods, but not freshwater fish. There are also small amounts in vegetables, dairy products and eggs. It is possible to develop an iodine deficiency, the most notable symptom being a swelling in the neck. This is usually a sign of thyroid enlargement—a treatable condition known as goiter and not uncommon. Iodized salt is salt to which iodine has been added. The RDA for iodine is 150 mcg, and eating fish twice a week should supply sufficient amounts.

Iron deficiency leads to anemia in many women until they are past childbearing age, after which dietary needs are lowered. However, the elderly may get too little from the diet, as may vegetarians. Foods rich in iron include red meat, liver, fish and eggs. There is also iron in cereals, fruits and vegetables, but less of it is absorbed. On the other hand, absorption is enhanced with vitamin C—so fresh fruits and green vegetables, which contain both, are important. Unprocessed bran and the tannin in tea and coffee make iron more difficult to absorb. Some breakfast cereals are fortified with extra iron—see the information on the outside of the box. The RDA for iron is 10 to 15 mg for adults other than pregnant women (who need more). A helping of beef supplies 3 mg of iron, fried liver 10 mg, a portion of cooked cabbage 0.36 mg, roast chicken 1 mg, and 1 slice whole-grain bread 1 mg.

Phosphorus plays a part in calcium absorption and formation of tissue between bones. We get it in meat, poultry fish, cereals, vegetables and soft drinks—but a diet high in carbonated drinks could provide too much phosphorus, interfering with calcium intake. The RDA for phosphorus is 800 to 1200 mg. A grilled steak contains 298 mg, a boiled egg 143 mg, a fresh tomato 16 mg, a portion of cooked cabbage 30 mg, and a large slice of bread 70 mg.

Potassium occurs plentifully in a variety of foods including instant coffee, meat, fish, bacon, dried fruit, bananas, green vegetables and milk. This mineral has a complementary action with sodium (found in salt), and many foods conveniently contain both. High sodium with low potassium intake is associated with high blood pressure. Loss of potassium can occur if large quantities of laxatives or diuretics (prescribed to reduce fluid retention) are taken and, in these cases, potassium supplements may be needed. Severe depletion of potassium may lead to heart failure but some people develop levels of potassium that are too high, a condition that can affect the heart and kidneys, meaning potassium-rich foods have to be reduced. There is no RDA for potassium, other than for pregnant and breastfeeding women. The U.K. Dietary Reference Value is 3500 mg. A medium potato contains 330 mg, a teaspoon of instant coffee 100 mg, a serving of cauliflower 144 mg, a portion of strawberries 190 mg, and a large slice of bread 70 mg.

Selenium is an antioxidant, and therefore part of the team of nutrients that fight damaging free radicals and protect against heart disease and cancer. Selenium deficiency in the soil was pinpointed as a possible reason for the high incidence of heart disease in Finland, where fertilizers are now enriched with the mineral. A report on diet in the Chinese province of Linxian (see "Vitamins Against Aging—No Doubt About It" earlier in this chapter) showed a 13 percent decline in the number of cancer deaths when selenium was given as part of a package of antioxidant supplements. Some research has shown that smokers have lower selenium levels than nonsmokers.

Most experts would say that we don't have to worry about getting enough selenium, and very high levels have been associated with an increased risk of heart disease. But we don't seem to take in very high levels, and we may have halved our intake in recent years. Selenium occurs in a variety of foods, including whole-grain bread, 100 g of which should supply the RDA average of 60 mcg. Cereals, liver, seafoods, red meat, chicken and eggs all contain selenium, though amounts vary with soil condition. Supplements may be combined with other antioxidants. There is some evidence that selenium is absorbed most efficiently when combined with zinc. A supplement should provide no more than 60 mcg of selenium.

Zinc deficiency has been recognized since the 1960s, mainly in connection with mental and physical retardation in adolescents, though it is also associated with hardening of the arteries, and with impotence. Zinc helps to neutralize the toxic mineral cadmium, high levels of which are associated with heart disease. Less than half the zinc in the diet is actually absorbed and certain foods interfere further with its absorption—unprocessed bran and whole-grain cereals containing phytic acid, as well as alcohol in large amounts. Some soil is depleted of zinc. The RDA for zinc is 12 to 15 mg, and the best sources of zinc are meat and some seafoods (oysters and crab). A quarter-pound grilled steak contains 6.8 mg, a helping of roast lamb 5 mg, a helping of beef stew 3 mg, 4 oysters 18 mg, and 3 large grilled sausages 2 mg. Sunflower, sesame and pumpkin seeds are also good sources of zinc, and there is some zinc in eggs and green leafy vegetables.

Chromium levels decline with age, strenuous exercise and a diet high in white sugar. This mineral helps to normalize blood sugar and cholesterol levels, and can correct sugar craving. It may also help to increase muscle mass. You can get it in liver, cheese, wheat germ and brewer's yeast. An uncontrollable sweet tooth may be a sign of lack of chromium in the diet. Sweet cravings occur when there are very low blood sugar levels. Eat something sweet and the blood sugar levels rise. Insulin is then produced to keep the levels under control. Without sufficient chromium, however, you don't get the insulin, and the sugar cravings remain. Some "alternative" nutritionists claim that a persistent sugar craving will be cured by taking a daily supplement of 10 to 150 mcg of chromium. The RDA for chromium is 50 to 200 mcg.

SWEET TOOTH SURVEY

A survey of women and sugar craving, carried out by Maryon Stewart of the Women's Nutritional Advisory Service, showed that high sugar consumption was linked with smoking, coffee drinking and eating less fresh fruit, vegetables and salad. Retired women consumed more sugar than women in any other group, including the unemployed. Those working as managers or directors consumed two-and-a-half times less. A taste for cakes, cookies and ice cream tended to increase with age; chocolate, soft drinks and alcohol tended to decrease. The cause of a sweet tooth could be a lack of chromium.

Calcium is important for men as well as women. Bone loss occurs with age in both sexes, though less severely in men unless they suffer from a condition that reduces calcium absorption. A diet high in protein can lead to excessive calcium excretion in the urine. Long-term use of steroids can also reduce absorption. See "Minerals for Menopause" earlier in this chapter for more on calcium.

THE ONE WE GET TOO MUCH OF

Sodium is an exception to the above list. A high intake of sodium is linked to an increased risk of high blood pressure, especially in people who are overweight and who drink a great deal of alcohol. Too much sodium may also be damaging for asthmatics. Sodium, a major constituent of salt, makes the air passages in the lungs more sensitive to irritants. Lung function improved in a group of asthmatics who switched to a low-salt diet, and deteriorated again when they returned to their former eating patterns.

It's not what we put into saucepans and on dinner plates that truly causes the problems. Salt added to processed foods contributes about 80 percent of the intake in many people's diets. The World Health Organization suggests that 4 g of salt daily is adequate for most needs. The average American consumes around 6 to 18 g a day.

Reading the contents of processed foods can help you cut sodium consumption. The 4 g daily salt allowance includes salt in cooking and in processed foods. One way to cut down on amounts in cooking and at the table is to block off half the holes in the salt shaker. Experiments with this revealed that those who remained free with the salt shaker did not even realize they were getting half portions of salt. Another suggestion is to use herbs and spices in place of salt and to cut down on processed food.

WHY FIBER IS ESSENTIAL

We tend to think of fiber in terms of breakfast cereals and whole-grain bread, but it's also found in fruits, vegetables, lentils and other legumes. Fiber is known to protect against coronary heart disease, bowel cancer and constipation. In Australia, where heart disease is at its lowest in over 40 years, fiber consumption is around 25 grams per person per day, and the Australian Nutrition Society is in no doubt of the link between those two facts.

What is not always made clear is which kinds of fiber offer which kinds of protection. Some components of high-fiber foods affect the large intestine only, some the small intestine and some both. Bowel cancer is the second main cause of cancer death in the industrial world, after lung cancer.

The rules about fiber are, in fact, fairly simple:

- **Cereal foods**—wheat, rice, corn, oats, rye and barley—differ from each other in their effects, and are the least soluble and most important sources of dietary fiber.

- **Legumes**—lentils, dried peas and beans—are more soluble.

- **Fruits and vegetables** are the most soluble, 50 to 60 percent, and are at least as important for their antioxidant properties as for fiber.

The best fiber for constipation and diverticular disease (weak pockets in the colon, causing muscle spasm and abdominal pain) is the insoluble variety. This creates bulk in the large bowel, is slow in fermenting and good at holding water, all qualities that keep the large bowel cell walls healthy. The bulk increases transit time and may also dilute any carcinogens in the intestine, thus reducing the risk of bowel cancer.

Wheat is the most insoluble source of dietary fiber. Rice is highly insoluble, too, but once the bran husk is milled off very little fiber remains, even in the brown variety. Pasta is usually wheat based and is more slowly digested than bread.

For **heart protection and lowering of cholesterol**, it's the effect fiber has on the small intestine that counts. Soluble and viscous dietary fiber slows the rate of absorption of glucose, aminoacids, cholesterol and fats.

Oats produce the best gummy, viscous fiber and have been shown to reduce cholesterol levels in those with already raised levels. The easiest way to eat this is in quick-cooking oatmeal. Barley is another source of viscous fiber. Rye is soluble, as are legumes, and they, too, have health-maintaining properties for the small intestine.

BIFIDUS, THE "FRIENDLY" BACTERIA

Yogurt, the long-time health-food favorite, has new scientific evidence to back up its claims. Bifidus, the so-called "friendly" bacteria found in the healthy intestine, can be enhanced by eating yogurt made with active bacteria.

Trials with bifidus-boosted yogurt by Professor Jean-Charles Grimaud in France have been shown to improve sluggish intestinal transit time in men and women volunteers. The effect was best for women, who may generally have a slower transit time than men. Professor Grimaud suggests that the yogurt could be a partial substitute for a high-fiber diet. Live "bio" or "bifidus" yogurts all contain active bacteria, but heating kills the beneficial properties.

HOW MUCH FIBER?

The average daily intake in the Western world is 12 g; the ideal dietary intake is 18 g. Here are the fiber contents of some common foods:

processed bran in breakfast cereals, 40 g serving	9.6 g
2 shredded wheat	5.5 g
helping of bran flakes *	3.9 g
helping of cornflakes	0.3 g
1 large slice whole-grain bread	3.4 g
white bread	1.1 g
serving of oatmeal	1.8 g
potato chips, small bag	3.5 g
2 medium boiled potatoes	2 g
small bag of peanuts	2 g
1 apple	2 g
100 g (4 oz) cooked lentils	4 g
100 g (4 oz) baked beans	8 g

*(Raw bran reduces iron and calcium absorption and is best avoided.)

We may never know how much of which type we actually need, since genetic makeup, lifestyle, length of intestine, stress responses, even components of individual meals, may vary the effect. Breakfast cereal bran is filling—and a good way to diet. When volunteers were given different

INCREASE YOUR FLUIDS

When nutritionist Carol Bateman, of London's Royal Free Hospital, persuaded her elderly patients to drink a minimum of half a gallon of fluid a day, she found that their constipation problems disappeared. Fortunately, this includes tea, coffee, fruit juice, soup, gravy and even the fluid in fruit, as well as water. As we age we lose body fluid from inside the cells rather than from tissue, and we need to consume extra to help flush the kidneys and reduce the risk of dehydration. High cereal-fiber diets retain fluid in the intestine and so extra is needed to compensate.

breakfasts either high in fiber, low in fiber, or only something to drink, by lunchtime the high-in-fiber breakfasters were able to eat considerably less than the other groups. This and other research confirms that fiber fills you up, making dieting easier. However, cereal fiber can cause gas and abdominal discomfort, especially in the first few weeks. Yogurt containing active bacteria may be taken as a partial substitute—see "Bifidus, the Friendly Bacteria" on page 55. And four to five slices of bread could provide enough fiber as a replacement for breakfast cereal.

THE PROTECTION OF FISH OILS

It doesn't sound too appetizing, but according to newspaper reports, bread containing fish oil is on sale in Denmark, and milk with fish oil is available in New Zealand. The reason behind this fishy additive is the enormous body of scientific evidence showing that fish-eating populations are less prone to heart disease and have longer life spans than populations where little fish is eaten. The Japanese and Eskimos, two cultures that enjoy high fish consumption, also enjoy low rates of heart disease.

Among the many medical trials, a recent one from Australia showed the effect of fish oil supplements on volunteers who were also given drugs that cause arteries to tense up and slow blood flow. Just 5 g of fish oils a day reduced the effect of the drugs by nearly a third, and higher doses wiped out two-thirds of the effect. A study in Wales in 1989 by the Medical Research Council revealed that men recovering from heart attacks reduced their risk of dying from another attack within the next two years by 29 percent when they ate high amounts of oil-rich fish.

There is no mystery about fish oils. They are known to contain essential fatty acids (EFAs); "essential" because the body cannot manufacture them, so they must be derived from the food we eat. The evidence suggests that they protect against heart disease, reduce blood pressure in those whose levels are raised, reduce inflammation associated with arthritis and skin conditions like psoriasis and may enhance the body's immune system.

The specific EFAs in fish oils are called omega-3. They can be converted into hormone-like substances called prostaglandins, which reduce the tendency of blood to clot, thus cutting the risk of heart attack. The reblocking of coronary arteries after angioplasty (a process that opens up a blocked artery by means of a small balloon attached to a catheter) has been found to be reduced when extra fish oil is included in the diet. Many trials demonstrate the effectiveness of fish oils in reducing raised blood pressure, but not in preventing this condition.

The effect on cholesterol levels is unclear, but omega-3 definitely lowers triglycerides, another type of fat found in the blood. Women at risk of heart disease may have low levels of cholesterol but a high level of triglycerides.

Another form of prostaglandin found in fish oils is thought to affect inflammatory conditions. Arthritis, caused by joint inflammation, and psoriasis, an inflammatory skin ailment, have been alleviated through fish oils. A study by Jill Belch at Ninewells Medical School in Scotland showed that patients with rheumatoid arthritis were able to reduce their painkillers by half after adding 5 to 10 g of fish oil to their daily diet. The 64 patients in the trial gained this relief in less than three months and retained it for the 15-month duration of the trial. This recent result backs up earlier findings of decreased joint pain with a daily intake of 15 to 20 g of cod liver oil. Improvements in psoriasis sufferers have also been mainly in the range of improvements, not cures, suggesting that fish oils are a valuable addition to other, more conventional treatments.

WHAT YOU CAN GET IN A CAPSULE

Fish oil supplements provide omega-3 if you don't want to think about diet, or if you don't need to push up amounts to help alleviate arthritis, etc. However, supplements in capsule form do not always provide adequate daily amounts of omega-3. Check on the package for contents; supplements should give 1 g omega-3 per day. A teaspoon of cod liver oil provides 0.85 g, but a cod liver oil capsule provides only 0.05 g, and halibut oil capsules provide even less.

REAL FISH OR FISH OIL SUPPLEMENTS?

If we're talking about prevention of heart disease, the question is easily answered. Drawing on current research, the suggested intake is 3.5 to 7 g of omega-3 a week. Mackerel supplies 3.5 g per 100 g helping, so one meal with mackerel per week, plus a second meal including any fish will do the trick. For arthritis or psoriasis relief, 5 to 10 g may be helpful. To reduce high blood pressure, 5 g may be effective.

Oil-rich fish has the most omega-3. It also contains a high level of vitamins A and D, which are good for skin and hair and contribute to the strengthening of bones. White fish and seafoods contain good back-up amounts.

Omega-3 content of fish per 100 g serving:

Mackerel		3.5 g
Salmon	*fresh*	2.7 g
	canned	1.7 g
	smoked	0.9 g
Herring		1.8 g
Sardine	*fresh*	2.1 g
	canned	1.7 g
Tuna	*fresh*	1.5 g
	canned	0.3 g
Cod		0.3 g
Haddock		0.3 g

CHOLESTEROL, FATTY FOODS AND THE MEDITERRANEAN DIET

HOW IMPORTANT ARE CHOLESTEROL LEVELS?

As the evidence for antioxidants as protection against heart disease gains ground, the case for antioxidants lowering cholesterol loses ground. A high level of cholesterol in the blood is a high risk factor for coronary heart disease, so reducing the level appears to make sense. But cholesterol levels are increasingly regarded as only one part of a complex picture that must also take into account body weight, amount of exercise, smoking and stress levels.

A few years ago, it was discovered that although fewer people died from heart disease when taking cholesterol-lowering drugs, the overall mortality rate among this group remained the same. Causes of death were such nondisease-related incidents as accidents, suicide and violence, so, bizarre as it may sound, there may be some hidden relation between low cholesterol levels and deaths from injury and suicide. One theory is that lowering cholesterol may increase aggressive or reckless behavior by creating an imbalance of a brain chemical called serotonin, which is associated with aggressive behavior.

Adding to the doubts is the finding that populations eating a diet that includes high amounts of polyunsaturated fats, instead of the cholesterol-forming saturated fats, do not enjoy a reduction in heart disease. It is now thought that the polyunsaturates themselves can increase cholesterol levels (see "Hydrogenated Oils—Going Easy on Polyunsaturates" later in this chapter.)

Long-term surveys of heart disease and the switch to low-fat diets are not showing the expected dramatic results that the theory behind low cholesterol demanded. Added to this is the finding that total serum cholesterol does not appear to be a strong predictor of coronary heart disease in people over 70. What counts in the elderly is the measure of certain "carriers" called low- and high-density lipoproteins (LDL and HDL) that determine the way cholesterol is transported through the bloodstream. And high levels of another fatty substance, triglyceride, are predictors of risk in women over 50 (see "Heart Disease and Women" in Chapter Three).

There is even a school of thought that says if you've made it into your 60s you've got good genes and can afford not to worry too much about coronary heart disease.

Undoubtedly, though, if members of your family haven't made it much past 60 and have died of heart disease, there is a very good chance that you've inherited a risk of abnormally high cholesterol levels, and need a carefully modified diet and possibly drug treatment to redress this.

Today, apart from this at-risk group, cholesterol gets a lower profile; however, we're by no means let off the hook where fat is concerned. All that the new approach means is that dietary cholesterol, derived from eggs and shellfish, can be eaten as it has a negligible effect on blood cholesterol. But fatty red meats, cheese, butter and cream need to be watched. There's still no escaping the fact that these animal fats are linked to high blood cholesterol and heart disease risk, as well as diabetes, obesity, high blood pressure and certain types of cancer. In people over 60, it can take about twice as long to remove dietary fat from the bloodstream than in younger people, probably because of reduced liver function. When the fat stays longer, there's a chance of more of it being deposited on the artery walls, thereby increasing narrowing of the arteries, a condition that can lead to heart disease. This is good reason to keep an eye on high-fat foods, especially meat.

VEGETARIANS LIVE LONGER

A study supported by the British Cancer Research Campaign looked at the mortality rates of meat eaters compared to nonmeat eaters over a period of 12 years. Death rates for meat eaters from all causes, including heart disease, were 54 percent of the national average, while it was 41 percent for vegetarians and fish eaters who ate meat less than once a week. Eating red meat five times or more a week exposes men to more than twice the risk of prostate cancer compared to men eating it only once a week, according to a study from the Harvard School of Public Health. Fortunately, the study also found that reducing red meat intake to three times a week could rapidly reduce the risk.

And more good news for vegetarians came out in 1994. A study of over 5000 vegetarians, over a period of 12 years, revealed that they had a 40 percent lower risk of dying of cancer and a 20 percent lower risk of dying of any cause when compared with 6000 carefully matched meat eaters. Vegetarians achieved this by eating cereals, legumes, fruits and vegetables, thus taking in less saturated fat and more antioxidants. The researchers, writing in the *British Medical Journal*, cautiously say, "Our data do not provide justification for encouraging meat eaters to change to a vegetarian diet. However, they do confirm that those who have chosen to do so might expect reductions in premature mortality due to cancer and possibly ischemic heart disease.

HOW THE MEDITERRANEAN DIET CUTS FATS

Countries such as France, Italy and Greece have lower rates of heart disease than do other Western countries. Hence the current popularity of the so-called Mediterranean diet, with evidence pointing to the good guy, olive oil, which is used for salads, cooking and as a dip with bread instead of butter. Mediterraneans also eat plenty of fruit, salads, bread, pasta (i.e., antioxidants and fiber), garlic (see the next section) and also wine (see "Drinking and Thriving" later in this chapter).

WALNUTS FOR A HEALTHY HEART

A study in the *New England Journal of Medicine* on eating walnuts suggests there's nothing like them for lowering cholesterol. One group of men were put on a normal healthy diet for four weeks and matched against another group who were given large amounts of walnuts in place of other fatty items. Both groups ended up with lower cholesterol, but that of the walnut eaters dropped by an extra 10 percent. Walnuts contain high levels of polyunsaturates, untainted by processing. About 25 g (1 oz) a week of walnut consumption is all that is needed.

A recent study from the French National Institute of Health and Medical Research showed the rapid effect of this diet. Half of 600 heart disease patients were asked to eat more bread, fish, poultry and vegetables, and less red meat, and to substitute margarine and olive oil for cream and butter. They also had to eat fruit every day and were allowed wine with meals. After two years they had suffered 70 percent fewer heart attacks than did patients who had continued with their usual diet.

A WHIFF OF GARLIC

Garlic can reduce cholesterol and discourage it from adhering to artery walls. Garlic may also be a potent cancer preventer, reducing tumors and attacking carcinogens that cause stomach cancer. And it can be a protection against food poisoning.

Is it essential to increase our garlic intake? The evidence to back up the claims about garlic is mixed. Fresh garlic has been shown to lower cholesterol levels, there's no doubt about that. It contains antibiotic, lipid (fat) lowering and detoxifying effects. But research and follow-up of garlic takers shows that you would need to devour at least seven cloves a day to lower cholesterol, and even then the effect may last only for several hours after intake. Many people would be allergic to this amount, and dermatitis, asthma and stomach irritation are associated with large amounts of garlic.

The alternative is to take commercial preparations, but contradictory results and poor research methods have drawn one team reviewing the evidence to the conclusion that "for this moment there is inadequate scientific justification for garlic supplementation." All the same, there is anecdotal evidence for reduced cholesterol levels in people taking garlic supplements. If your cholesterol levels need reducing, choose a reputable brand from health food shops and check out the results.

FATS FOR COOKING AND EATING— WHICH TO CHOOSE

TYPES OF FAT

Oils for cooking and spreading are composed of saturated, polyunsaturated and monounsaturated fatty acids.

- **Saturated fats,** such as butter, cheese, lard and the fat on red meat, are solid at room temperature, and most are derived from animals. In addition, ordinary margarine contains saturated fats, though not as much as butter. And two vegetable oils are classed as saturates: coconut and palm oil. These are the villains where cholesterol is concerned.

- **Polyunsaturates** are usually liquid at room temperature or when chilled. They are vegetable oils—corn, sunflower, safflower, soya, grapeseed and walnut—and also the omega-3 kind of oil found in fish (see page 57). The latest thinking on polyunsaturates is that one can be too liberal with them—see the facts about hydrogenated oils, below.

- **Monounsaturates** are usually liquid at room temperature but may solidify if chilled. Vegetable oils classed as monounsaturates are olive, hazelnut, rapeseed, groundnut and many blended vegetable oils. This is what the Mediterranean diet is about.

Cut the unhealthy fat by avoiding the saturates, which can be achieved by trimming the fat off meat, choosing poultry instead of red meat, avoiding the use of shortening and lard, and substituting nonfat yogurt for sour cream. Buy low-fat spreads instead of butter or margarine, but check that they are low in saturates, and if you are watching your weight, remember that polyunsaturate doesn't mean lower in calories. Cakes, cookies and other desserts have hidden fat, not to mention sugar, so save these for special occasions and get sweetness from fresh, stewed and dried fruits instead. Be stingy with the sugar when cooking.

Also, there are the benefits of lean cooking: grill, bake with foil covering, broil or steam instead of frying. Use a minimum amount of oil and nonstick pans, and avoid batter and breadcrumb coatings. Choose nonfat (skim) or 1-percent low-fat milk rather than whole milk.

The best of the monounsaturates is olive oil, either top-grade extra virgin oil or the refined and blended standard oil. For a cheaper alternative, go for rapeseed oil or blended vegetable oils.

HYDROGENATED OILS—
GOING EASY ON POLYUNSATURATES

If you read the labels on many margarines and processed foods such as cookies and chips, you are likely to come across the term "hydrogenated vegetable oils." This hydrogenating processing makes the oils firmer at room temperature and gives them a longer shelf life. Unfortunately, it also increases levels of trans fatty acids, yet another substance present in saturated fats, oils and fatty foods. Too much trans fatty acid can make blood cholesterol rise as much as saturated fats do. And the trans fatty acid content of these processed polyunsaturates is often higher than in saturates. This comparatively recent finding may be the key to

FEAR OF FRYING

When oxygen meets oil at high temperature, the result can be oxidized fatty acids, which contain those damaging free radicals. Also, the vitamin E content of fats, a known antioxidant, is destroyed through heat. The rule here is to not reuse oil from deep frying, especially if it tastes odd—it probably means the oil is rancid, a sign of oxidation. Don't reuse cooking oil or fat after shallow frying—the oxidizing effect is even stronger. Monounsaturates are less prone to oxidation than other fats. Always store cooking oils in cupboards, so they are not exposed to sunlight, another oxidizing agent.

---

persistently high death rates from heart disease in populations that consume large amounts of polyunsaturates.

Confused and perplexed by now? So are the experts. Try following these guidelines:

- If you eat a high-polyunsaturate margarine or other spread instead of butter, limit it to go on four slices of bread a day, maximum. Use olive oil or another monounsaturate for cooking and in salad dressings, not polyunsaturate cooking oil.

- Since the trans fatty acid in butter is actually less than in many processed substitutes, you might consider putting butter on bread, in modest amounts, instead. Or there's always the Italian way—stick to the monounsaturates and dip your bread into olive oil.

- Watch those cookies, cakes and other store-bought desserts for their hydrogenated oil content. You can often identify them from ingredients lists on labels—look out for "hydrogenized edible oil" and "partially hydrogenated vegetable oils."

- We need some fat in our diet, but far less than most of us get. Around 100 g per day for a man, and 70 g for a woman is a healthy level. Many people take in twice that amount. Though it is not easy to measure intake, try a rough assessment for a few days by writing down the estimated fat content of the foods you eat.

DRINKING AND THRIVING

ALCOHOL—WHAT THEY'RE SAYING NOW

The French are a case in point. They certainty smoke too much, may eat fatty foods like cheese, and may cook with butter, yet they have lower rates of coronary heart disease than many other Western populations. It's the red wine of course. Most of us have heard the good news: moderate regular drinking of wine, especially red wine, is beneficial to your health. It is claimed to cut coronary thrombosis by 40 percent and stroke by 25 percent, it has been found to reduce the bone-thinning effects of aging and osteoporosis in middle-aged men as well as women, and may even stop the onset of some cancers and dementia.

Wine drinking is very much part of the Mediterranean diet, which is full of heart-protecting monounsaturates (i.e., olive oil), fiber, fish and plentiful vegetables. However, growing evidence gives the go-ahead for alcohol, especially in the form of red wine, to be taken in moderation on a regular basis.

But what about the effect of alcohol on aging—is it bad for the digestive system, does it kill off brain cells? Until recently, nobody gave much thought to alcohol and the elderly, except in a spoilsport sort of way, indicating that it must be more of a risk than to younger people, and should be taken in even smaller quantities.

According to Oliver James, Professor of Geriatric Medicine at the University of Newcastle upon Tyne in England, healthy 70 year olds filter alcohol out of their systems just as quickly as 35 year olds. The liver, it seems, does not age greatly with the years. The red-veined noses and flushed older faces associated with heavy alcohol consumption are due to an intermediate substance called acetaldehyde caused by the way some people metabolize alcohol. But remember, drinking in moderation may be good for you. Drinking in excess is certainly the route to liver disease.

As for the brain cells, there's no evidence to show that moderate drinking contributes to Alzheimer's disease. On the contrary, in a study of

241 elderly patients registered with London general practitioners that assessed alcohol consumption, cognitive impairment and depression, no association was shown between drinking and depression, falls or the need for medical treatment. Among the men studied, it was the nondrinkers who were more likely to show cognitive impairment.

> *Beer is rich in silicon, a mineral that can mop up harmful aluminum. Since aluminum may be linked with Alzheimer's disease, it could be a useful protection.*

A study from Boston of low-to-moderate drinkers and smokers, aged from 65 to 80-plus, again showed no cognitive impairment. In this study, the 1201 men and women were checked twice over a three-year span. Other investigations have revealed that elderly drinkers who have just one drink a week scored significantly better in memory tests than nondrinkers.

Professor Oliver James maintains that recent or lifelong abstinence from alcohol is associated with a higher risk of stroke and that moderate consumption is therefore somehow protective. That protection could be in the form of reducing the risk of blood clotting. A report in *Pulse* magazine of a meeting held by the American College of Cardiologists in Wisconsin told of how two or three glasses of red wine could, within half an hour, reduce blood-clotting time by 8 percent.

The evidence collected by Professor James was based on a study of patients admitted to Newcastle hospitals suffering from stroke, compared to a second matched group of 650 individuals who had not suffered a stroke. All were questioned on their drinking habits. Over the two-year period monitored, there were more stroke victims in the teetotalers than in the moderate drinkers, a finding confirmed by other studies in the United States.

Professor James recommends a small drink in the evening as an excellent night sedative for elderly people (and no doubt for those in middle age, as well).

And a final recommendation comes from a French homeopathic doctor, Emmeric Maury, who has extolled the virtues of drinking red wine moderately with every meal, a habit which, he said, could help alleviate gastric problems, obesity, arthritis, constipation and even cellulite, depending on the grape and quality of the wine. Dr. Maury died at age 87, a fact which could help prove his point.

For all these discoveries, including the bad news for teetotalers, there are still puzzles and question marks. Some studies provide different conclusions. One of the biggest, and most difficult to ignore, comes from Norway where the incidence of cancer in 5332 teetotalers was compared with that of the whole population from the years 1980 to 1989. Kristina Kjaerheim, of the Institute of Epidemiological Cancer Research in Oslo, found 350 new cases of cancer in the nondrinking group compared to an expected rate of 478 derived from the general population. That meant a dramatic difference of 27 percent. A sobering thought, but one to comfort many who have given up drinking, especially those in the 50-plus age group.

MODERATE OR MEAN-SPIRITED?

Moderate drinking means 14 units for women and 21 for men—a unit being 8 oz of beer, a glass of wine or a small shot of hard liquor—best spread out over a week, with perhaps a day or two off except for the nightcap. However, there is growing evidence that these limits, at least for men, may be unnecessarily low, and that something in the region of 29 units a week could be recommended. Women are at greater risk of liver disease and breast cancer through alcohol, possibly because female stomachs contain less of an enzyme that breaks down alcohol, and there is no research so far to suggest a change in safety limits.

TEA, COFFEE, AND A LOT OF DON'T KNOWS

Here it comes again—another protection against heart disease. This time it's instant coffee, with five or more cups a day linked to reduced heart disease in 10,000 men and women surveyed in Scotland. Coffee drinking may also improve reaction times, verbal memory and reasoning ability, if a survey of over 9000 adults is anything to go by, and tea drinking may do the same.

However, brewed coffee has been associated with raising cholesterol levels and with higher risk of heart disease (the instant kind is weaker and contains less caffeine than do beans). Brewing ground coffee may release certain harmful chemicals, and to make things even grimmer, the chlorine bleach in filter papers is suspected of being carcinogenic. The evidence is mixed and contradictory on these findings. An overview of 11 different recent research papers actually clears real coffee of its potential dangers. Meanwhile, bypass the problem and use unbleached coffee filters. Keep a top limit of five cups a day, and bear in mind the following findings:

- Caffeine can constrict blood vessels and cause headaches, increase jitteriness, irritability, heartburn, premenstrual tension and menopausal hot flashes. And it may possibly contribute to infertility.

- Two or more cups of coffee a day reduces bone density in women. However, the balance can be somewhat redressed by also drinking at least one glass of milk a day, according to a report from the *Journal of the American Medical Association*.

- Despite these effects, it is not true that coffee should be avoided by people with raised blood pressure. Reports suggest that caffeinated and decaffeinated coffee have no significant effect on blood pressure. Caffeine at the end of a meal, when given to healthy elderly people, has prevented dizziness by stopping a sudden postprandial fall in blood pressure.

- Is caffeine connected with benign fibrocystic breast disease? Earlier evidence in the 1980s said yes, later evidence says no. There is some indication that giving up coffee reduces breast nodules, but any changes are not considered significant.

- A cup of decaffeinated coffee yields about 3 mg of caffeine, compared with 100 to 150 mg from coffee made with ground beans. The "Swiss water process," which uses pure water and carbon filters is said to be the safest method of taking out the caffeine. Even so, decaf may be bad for you. A high consumption could moderately increase the risk of heart disease—research has shown that it raises cholesterol levels. Limit your intake to 3 to 4 cups a day.

- The caffeine content of a cup of tea is 20 to 50 mg. But on the other hand, tea too may guard against heart disease. It contains flavonoids, a natural chemical that inhibits buildup of fatty deposits in the arteries and mops up free radicals.

Perhaps the safest thing to do is to give up coffee and switch to noncaffeine herbal teas, now available in a wide range of flavors. Or wait until a newly developed natural noncaffeine bean is made available.

SMOKE SCREENS

You can't smoke and age successfully at the same time. Two packs of cigarettes a day are said to increase the risk of heart disease 20 times. Lung cancer and respiratory ailments are also greater risks, as well as bladder cancer, and there's the likelihood of an earlier than average menopause and prematurely lined skin. Even women who are passive smokers—who live with heavy smokers—tend to experience earlier menopause.

WAYS TO BREAK THE SMOKING HABIT

There's no sure way to stop smoking. You have to find a method that suits you best. Here are a few tried and tested methods:

Stopping cold. You have to make the decision positively in your mind before you fix a date and stick to it.

Aversion therapy. Again, pick a stop date and then, for the two days before it, smoke four times as many cigarettes as you normally would—ideally to the point where you can't stand the thought of any more. You can even try a stronger variety than normal to accentuate the distaste, chain-smoking if you can. Then retire for the night and give up completely next morning. Don't go for this method if you have any medical condition that could be exacerbated by smoking.

The on-off approach. Try giving up for a day or two as a test period. If you find you can do it, repeat the giving-up for a week. When you feel sufficiently confident, make the giving-up time permanent.

Switching and swapping. Change brands, smoke using the hand you normally don't use. Smoke at unusual times and never when you normally would do so. Don't smoke where you usually do—in restaurants, or while watching television perhaps. Do smoke in places you normally don't—maybe the bathroom or bedroom (but not in bed). After two or three weeks of this, set yourself a day for quitting completely.

Cutting down gradually. Reduce daily, setting a period of two weeks or a month until you get down to no smoking at all. Smoke half a cigarette only, don't inhale or try using cigarette substitutes to replace normal cigarettes.

Get outside help. Join a self-help group. Talking to others may make it easier for you to recognize your vulnerable moments and to strengthen your resolve. Or try hypnotherapy—not a magical cure, but effective for some people as a method of curbing their addiction.

Nicotine substitutes. Giving up is easier with the help of a nicotine patch, which causes peak levels of nicotine to form in the brain within a couple of hours. A nasal spray delivers the nicotine to the brain within minutes. These products may not reduce dependency, however, and some health professionals are coming to the conclusion that these aids may have to be used as permanent substitutes.

Some substitutes themselves could increase the risk of heart disease if used for long periods, according to Professor Colin Caro of the Centre for Biological and Medical Systems at Imperial College, London. Ultrasound scans have shown temporary stiffening of the artery wall of non-smokers after they have chewed nicotine gum, and Professor Caro suggests that anyone who already has a heart condition should not chew the gum for a long period of time. Nicotine may stimulate a release of adrenalin which makes the heart beat faster and arteries become stiffer.

Low-tar cigarettes may increase craving rather than curb it. People have been found to simply smoke more. Lowest-tar cigarettes may slightly reduce the risk of lung cancer, but offer no protection from other conditions associated with smoking.

SUMMING UP—
GUIDELINES FOR THE BEST POSSIBLE DIET

TWELVE GOLDEN RULES

1. Eat vegetables and salads daily. The best diet is a combination of green, leafy vegetables, yellow and orange vegetables, peas and beans for fiber content and uncooked salads. Eat at least three helpings a day.

2. Have two to four servings of fresh fruit daily.

3. Go for fiber. You'll get it in cereals, and it's a way to make calcium-rich milk go down, too, so try to eat at least one helping a day. Other fiber foods that can protect against heart disease and bowel disorders are bananas, avocados, celery, fresh fruit, lentils and other dried beans and legumes, and oatmeal.

4. Limit meat consumption. Red meat is best kept to two to three helpings a week; substitute chicken, fish and nuts as sources of protein.

5. Eat fish at least twice a week, including some of the oil-rich varieties such as herring, mackerel and sardines.

6. Limit fats and dairy products. Use olive, sunflower or safflower oils rather than animal fats for cooking, and grill, bake, braise, boil and steam instead of frying. Reduce oils and fats by using nonstick pans. Choose skim milk, low-fat "live" yogurts and cottage cheese, and low-fat hard cheeses. Remember monounsaturated fats, such as olive and rapeseed oil, are healthiest.

7. Drink plenty of liquid. It can be water, up to six large glasses daily, fruit juice or herbal tea, which is, of course, caffeine-free.

8. Cut down on caffeine, don't boil coffee beans, limit decaffeinated coffee to three to four cups a day.

9. Alcohol consumption should be limited. The maximum safe limit for women is 14 units a week, and for men 21 units are recommended: one unit is 8 ounces of beer, a small glass of wine or a standard shot of hard liquor.

10. Reduce sugar, not only in tea and coffee, but by choosing natural, unsweetened fruit juice instead of soft drinks. And don't forget the sugar content of cakes, cookies and jams. Try fresh fruit for dessert instead.

11. Reduce salt, both in cooking and when seasoning food at the table. Some salted foods you need to keep under control are chips, salted nuts, smoked fish, bacon, smoked and cured meats like salami and ham, pickles and bottled sauces like soy sauce. Have these no more than two to three times a week.

12. Don't smoke.

> *The effect of fish oil capsules and garlic tablets, or other special dietary supplements, is small compared with the effect of changing your overall diet, getting exercise and quitting smoking, says Dr. Mark Rayner of the Coronary Prevention Group.*

VITAMINS AND MINERALS—THE COMPLETE LIST

Some of these figures represent estimated safe maximum intake. Figures here are for adults and elderly only, not for pregnant or breast-feeding women.

Recommended Daily Allowances (RDAs)

Vitamins	RDAs
Vitamin A as beta-carotene	2666–3333 IU
Retinol equivalent	800–1000 mcg
Vitamin B_1	1.0–1.5 mg
Vitamin B_2	1.2–1.7 mg
Vitamin B_6	1.6–2 mg
Vitamin B_{12}	2.0 mcg
Vitamin C	60 mg
Vitamin D_2	200–400 IU
Vitamin D_2	5–10 mcg
Vitamin E	8–10 mg
Vitamin K_1	50–60 mcg
Biotin	30–100 mcg
Nicotinamide	15–19 mg
Pantothenic acid	4–7 mg
Folic acid	180–200 mcg

Minerals and Trace Elements	RDAs
Calcium	800–1200 mg
Iron	10–15 mg
Copper	1.5–3.0 mg
Magnesium	280–350 mg
Zinc	12–15 mg
Iodine	150 mcg
Manganese	2.5 mg
Potassium	2000–3500 mg
Phosphorus	800–1200 mg
Selenium	55–70 mcg
Chromium	50–200 mcg
Molybdemum	75–250 mcg

CHAPTER THREE

The Challenge of Staying Healthy

TRACKING DOWN THE AGING GENES

A healthy lifestyle can't guarantee a trouble-free old age. Some people are unlucky enough to get lung cancer without ever having touched a cigarette; moderate drinkers can develop liver disease; athletes, non-smokers and low-fat eaters can be struck down by a heart attack; and even yoga teachers have been known to have hip replacements.

To some extent we can't escape our personal vulnerabilities, especially those we have inherited. We all carry potentially harmful genes, and many illnesses, including cancer, heart disease and even mental illness, may be influenced by our genetic makeup. But on the horizon are major advances that could change all this, and the horizon is very near.

Within the next 15 years, geneticists working on the Human Genome Project will have perfected tests capable of revealing around 1000 inherited illnesses. In some cases we can look forward to therapies that will correct defective genes. In other cases, knowing our potential physical weaknesses may give us the incentive to follow a healthy lifestyle and diet. And regular monitoring of anyone known to be at risk will provide a greater opportunity to treat, and maybe cure, a disease in its early stages.

The American Academy of Anti-Aging Medicine, launched in the autumn of 1993, claims to be the first medical society recognizing reversibility of the aging process. At the inauguration, one of its members, Vincent Giampapa, talked of biomarkers, clinical tests that will soon provide measurement of the aging status of patients, in the form of cellular, molecular and chromosomal information.

Scientists are envisioning a time when we will all carry "genetic passports" showing which diseases we are vulnerable to. This genetic information could be based on simple saliva tests, possibly bought over the counter like home pregnancy tests. However, this prospect is not entirely rosy. We may come to live in a society in which abortion and invitro fertilization are used on a large scale to screen out defects, and insurance companies and employers might insist on gene testing before taking on clients or staff. Smokers who find that they are not susceptible to lung cancer may have something to celebrate, but not prospective lung cancer victims who will suffer through passive smoking unless we find means of genetic repair or more effective treatments. Already, some women with a family history of breast or ovarian cancer are opting for surgical removal even when there are no signs of disease.

Over and above everything else, we are facing a profound shift toward preventive medicine in the not-too-distant future, much of it being the fitness-and-nutrition kind described earlier in this book, but with targeting of specific individuals who will know their personal risks.

For the present, almost every week brings news of yet another gene being identified. Scientists are tracking down a defective gene for breast and ovarian cancer, so soon women known to be vulnerable will be distinguished from others unaffected by their family history. A gene for colon cancer has been isolated, and this condition is curable if detected early. The gene for Huntington's disease, which strikes in middle age and causes lack of coordination and ultimately dementia, was identified in 1993. Scientists are now looking for a gene for atherosclerosis, and have already detected a substance called PAI-1, high levels of which prevent the breakdown of blood clots, leading to a narrowing of the arteries and the risk of heart attack and stroke. And one of the most promising discoveries is a genetic factor that seems to cause heart attacks in nonsmoking people of normal weight, with normal blood pressure and normal blood-fat levels.

> *Imagine a time when you might be offered an injection containing a cocktail of anti-aging genes. Perhaps we might get them in infancy, like vaccinations, or as boosters throughout out life in the form of injections or even a nasal spray.*

We are also at the start of a major new way to treat disease. Gene therapy, methods that target cells of affected organs, are already making their mark. Around 50 different lines of treatment had been approved in the United States as of mid-1993. One treatment developed in the United Kingdom is already saving lives of children with enzyme-deficiency conditions, and trials are planned for gene repair of people with cystic fibrosis. Cancer cells may be destroyed via supplies of tumor-suppressor genes or cells that activate the immune system, and these methods, possibly given by injection or in pill form, are expected to become as routine as chemotherapy and radiation therapy. There's even hope that a gene for the healthy blood fat known as LDL may be given to people with inherited high-cholesterol levels.

The prospects get even better. Imagine a time when you might be offered an injection containing a cocktail of anti-aging genes. Perhaps we might get them in infancy, like vaccinations, or as boosters throughout our life in the form of injections or even a nasal spray.

Such gene intervention would not fight specific conditions, but would tackle the basic process of aging itself. The discoveries described in the previous pages concern illnesses, some of them chronic diseases, associated with aging. But chronic diseases are not a necessary adjunct to aging. Some people enjoy a very long life span without contracting any of them. What we all do in time, however, is succumb to the aging process, i.e., the gradual deterioration of bodily function. The long-term Baltimore Longitudinal Study of Aging, begun in 1958, is observing more than 1000 people aged from 20 to over 90, and is pointing the way to a new understanding of the aging process.

What is becoming apparent is that there are great variations in the way individuals age, with different organs in an individual aging at different rates. Several distinct processes are involved, and genes, plus lifestyle, plus diseases, affect the rate of aging.

The American National Institute on Aging is funding important work in this area. Dr. Thomas Johnson at the University of Colorado in Boulder has altered a gene in the roundworm and increased its maximum life span by 110 percent. Dr. Michal Jazwinski, at the Louisiana State University Medical Center in New Orleans, has found genes that extend the period of activity in yeast by 30 percent and enabled it to continue dividing for up to 28 generations, rather than the usual 21 cell divisions. And there is the well-publicized, long-lived fruit fly, whose life span was nearly doubled through genetic selection in the laboratory of Michael Rose at the University of California, Irvine.

The genes isolated for these experiments are only a few of what may be hundreds of longevity-related genes, and scientists are now trying to find whether there are counterparts in humans.

GENES IN ACTION

Another aim is to identify what the genes involved in these experiments actually do.

Gene products in the form of proteins carry out many important functions in cells and body tissue that appear to affect aging. The antioxidant enzyme superoxide dismutase, otherwise known as SOD, for instance, seems to prevent cell damage. This finding supports the theories about diet and the effect of antioxidants on free radicals, described in Chapter Two.

Other gene products are thought to control cell senescence, the stage at which cells stop dividing. Cell division is reduced with age, and how the process works at this level is still a mystery, involving intricate mechanisms and interactions. An understanding of this could also lead to a greater understanding of cancer, which is caused by cells that escape the control mechanisms.

Glycation, or **glucose crosslinking**, is a new research area connected with cell deterioration. Glucose molecules attach themselves to proteins, triggering a set of crosslinking processes and end products (called AGEs). These products may cause age-related changes and conditions such as diabetes. The body has a defense system against crosslinking, though it becomes less efficient as we age. Diabetes researchers are looking at ways to block AGE formation with drugs.

DNA, the generic information system necessary for all cellular function, suffers damage from free radicals and other toxic agents. In time, this damage leads to malfunctioning and ultimately to deterioration of tissues and organs. But to compensate, numerous enzyme systems in the cell have evolved to try to repair the damage. Humans repair DNA more efficiently than mice or other short-lived animals, which could be a reason why we live longer. What gerontologists are finding is that repair rates vary among cells, and that the most efficient repair goes on at the very start of human life, in sperm and egg cells.

Heat shock proteins (HSP) are substances produced as a response to stress, and they decline with age, which is why researchers are interested in them. Old animals placed under stress, such as unnatural physical restraint, have lower levels of an HSP named HSP-70. This also declines in laboratory cultures of aging cells. HSPs seem to help repair and replace damaged cells and, although little more is known about them at present, they may turn out to be linked with growth hormones and could throw light on factors in the aging process.

Growth hormones offer one of the more dramatic advances in this field. A small group of men aged 60 and over at Veteran Administration hospitals in Milwaukee and Chicago received injections of synthetic growth hormone (GH) for a short period of time. GH is produced in the pituitary gland, and plays a critical part in normal growth and development in childhood. It may also have a role in aging, which the experiment seems to confirm. The injections, three times a week, dramatically reversed certain aging signs: lean body mass and muscle increased; skin became thicker; excess body fat was reduced. When the injections stopped, middle-aged spread, thinning of skin and reduced muscle power returned.

We make less GH as we get older, a development linked with excess abdominal fat. Obesity depresses production of GH while exercise encourages it. Unfortunately, regular injections of GH would be trading in a trim waistline for more serious problems: long-term GH therapy is associated with an increased risk of heart disease and diabetes.

Other hormones also play a part in aging. The sex hormones estrogen and testosterone both decline with age, and given as therapy they can increase bone strength and provide other benefits (see "Menopause and After" later in this chapter). Certain hormones that appear to decline in humans from about the age of 30 may be connected with the immune system and chronic diseases, offering much to excite and engage researchers in this new territory.

The rest of this chapter looks at chronic conditions and illnesses associated with aging, and at the newest techniques regarding predicting and screening for disease, and protecting against it.

HEARTS AND INHERITANCE

Over the last quarter century, the number of deaths from heart disease in the United States and Australia has fallen by about 50 percent, which may be due to effective health education on the roles of smoking, exercise and diet.

Men under 65 are more than three times as likely to develop a heart condition as women, although premenopausal protection disappears as women get older. Only in the last few years have researchers begun to realize that what applies to men often has little bearing on women. Men in low-level jobs are three times more at risk than executives, the poor more than the affluent. One of the most commonly performed surgical techniques in the Western world is coronary bypass to correct the effect of blocked arteries.

The risk factors for heart disease are high cholesterol, elevated blood pressure, smoking, diabetes, hereditary factors and stress. Obesity is only considered a risk in men if there are other factors, but is a significant risk in women. Body shape can be predictive, with men and women who are thick at the waist most at risk because of the kind of fat found there (see Chapter Four). Men with severe baldness on the crown of the head are three times more at risk than men with full hair, a finding that has been linked with an enzyme's effect on the male sex hormone testosterone. All these factors can be reduced by a healthy lifestyle.

Bacteria have also been linked to heart disease—a chronic stomach infection in childhood is one condition associated with an increased risk of coronary heart disease in later life, although the research is too new to draw any firm conclusions.

CHOLESTEROL

This well-known substance is a waxy compound produced by the body and also derived from food. It is not all bad, being necessary for cell composition, hormone production and digestion of dietary fat. We get most

---

HOW TO RECOGNIZE A HEART ATTACK OR STROKE

Pain in the chest is not the only sign of a heart attack. Recognizing signs and getting the victim to a hospital as soon as possible can be the difference between life and death. Look for:

- intense pain in center of chest; may spread to arms
- shortness of breath, sweating, skin pallor
- fainting or feeling of weakness
- nausea, vomiting

A stroke may include the above symptoms, but does not include pain. The other main symptoms of a stroke are numbness, often on one side of the body, difficulty in speaking or in understanding speech, loss of vision in one eye, dizziness and loss of balance.

of it, a good 80 percent, from eating saturated fats in the form of fatty meat, butter and cheese, which are converted to cholesterol. The rest, the amount our bodies make for us, comes mainly from the liver, the skin and the small intestine.

Ideas about cutting down cholesterol are changing as research is beginning to show that for most people it is not in itself a good predictor of heart-disease risk. But before recent doubts set in, the theory was as follows: When too much cholesterol is consumed, or when the body cannot process it properly, cholesterol accumulates in the blood, leaving deposits that clog the arteries and slow down blood flow to the heart. This condition, atherosclerosis, can lead to blood clotting, heart attacks and strokes.

Nowadays, the focus is on "carriers" called lipoproteins, which transport cholesterol in the blood. Low-density lipoproteins (LDLs) do the dirty work, depositing cholesterol in the artery walls. When doctors talk about high levels of LDL, it is not good news. High-density lipoproteins (HDLs) are another story. They carry cholesterol away from the artery walls into the liver, where the body can excrete it. It is plainly beneficial to have high levels of HDL. (If you want to remember the good from the bad, try thinking of H for "healthy" and L for "lethal.")

In people over 70, these "carriers" serve as better predictors of heart disease than do cholesterol levels. Dr. Scott Grundy, speaking at the British Hyperlipidaemia Association annual conference in 1993, suggested that with aging there is a natural decline in receptors that attract LDLs and HDLs. These receptors are on the cell surfaces of the liver, and the fewer the HDLs, the less chance there is of clearing cholesterol from the blood.

Older people who exercise regularly are the exception to this rule. For them, their cholesterol level does seem to reflect their health status, just as it does in the younger population, according to an investigation of over 2000 people aged from 65 to 74 published in the *Journal of the American Geriatrics Society*. Perhaps this is because exercise can enhance HDL levels and possibly also their receptors, though more research is needed so confirm this.

Blood-cholesterol levels are not constant. They can go up and down in any given individual. This may be one reason why over-the-counter cholesterol-testing kits are so notoriously unreliable, and why even laboratory equipment is not totally accurate. A study published in *Hospital Doctor* revealed a consistent 4-percent overestimation error, which doubled the number of patients who appeared to need drugs. The researchers also found that smokers with high blood pressure were four times more likely to die from heart disease than nonsmokers with low blood pressure *but with the same cholesterol levels*. They conclude that quitting smoking and taking half an aspirin daily will do more for most people with high cholesterol than drugs will, with the exception of those who have inherited the condition.

SOME PEOPLE ARE BORN WITH HIGH CHOLESTEROL LEVELS

Cutting down on cholesterol may no longer be the mainstream way to reduce heart disease, but it is still essential for people who are born with high levels due to an inherited lack of "good" receptors. If a family member has a heart attack before the age of 45, it's a sign that other family members could be diagnosed with familial hypercholesterolemia (FH). Some other signs include xanthomas, cholesterol deposits that take the form of yellow raised "lumps" on the knuckles or on the Achilles tendon, a white ring round the iris and yellow fat deposits around the eye or lid. Treatment for people with FH consists of prescription medications and a specialized diet.

CHOLESTEROL LEVELS— WHAT THEY CAN TELL YOU ABOUT YOUR HEALTH

Findings such as those above are casting doubts on the value of testing cholesterol levels, though medical opinions differ. In the United States, recommendations include testing adults every five years, and there is an increasing interest in monitoring HDL and LDL levels in high-risk individuals. The British Heart Foundation states that "measurement of cholesterol levels may only be necessary when there are other risk factors noted. These include smoking, family history, obesity and high blood pressure." There are many variables to take into account: cholesterol levels increase with age, vacillate with the menstrual cycle and go sky-high during pregnancy.

Desirable cholesterol levels should be below **5.2 millimoles per liter of blood** for men. The research on safe levels for women is still in its infancy, but there is a growing belief that they can tolerate higher levels. This may also be true of older people of both sexes, so that the middle category below may represent acceptable levels for those aged 70 and over.

- At **5.2 to 6.5** millimoles per liter you have a moderate risk, which is increased through smoking, lack of exercise, stress and a family history of heart disease. A change of diet and more exercise could be all that's needed.

- At **6.5 to 7.8** you need to talk to your doctor, who should give you three to six months to see results from diet changes, plus perhaps some further investigation. If there is no change, medications to lower cholesterol may be needed.

- At **over 7.8** you likely have an inherited problem, and medical supervision with drugs will be needed.

HOW OUR PAST PREDICTS
THE WAY WE GROW OLD

From 1911 onward, every baby born in the English county of Hertfordshire was weighed at birth, seen regularly by a health visitor during the first year and weighed again when one year old. In 1992 Professor David Barker was able to publish some extraordinary findings based on the still-preserved records of this practice. He traced the men, around 6000 of them, born in one part of the county during 1911 to 1930, and found that some still survived. Those who had weighed 18 pounds or less at the age of one year were three times as likely to have died from heart disease by the age of 65 as babies who had weighed 27 pounds. Death rates fell progressively with increasing weight at one year of age. Stroke fatalities followed this pattern too.

There were similar, though less strong, trends with a low birth weight of 6.5 pounds or less. Men who had a small head circumference and were thin at birth had a greater risk of dying from heart disease before the age of 65 than fatter, bigger-headed babies. Low birth weight was also associated with raised blood pressure and diabetes in later life.

READING PALMS

Fingertip and palm patterns can predict the future in terms of blood pressure. And it's all there from birth. Certain whorls, palm prints, and even hand shape and size (for example, long, slim right hands) in babies are associated with raised blood pressure in adult life. The vulnerable signs were found in babies who were long and slim or shorter than average at birth, already identified as candidates for the condition. Fingertip whorls are determined by the 19th week of pregnancy; so might be future high blood pressure.

Other findings are equally sensational. Low-weight babies with big placentas, a combination indicating that the fetus was starved and stressed in early pregnancy, were at risk for later high blood pressure. A second group of babies, traced from records in another county that are similar to the Hertfordshire ones, also developed high blood pressure in later life. These babies were average in weight at birth, but below average in length, i.e., 20 inches or less.

These findings persist regardless of social class, smoking, alcohol consumption and obesity, judging from the surviving men in the surveys. The research is thought to be similar for women (tracing women born 70 years ago was not so easy, since many changed their names through marriage). The conclusion at present is that there is a critical period before birth when blood pressure is sensitive to programming, and a period up to one year after the birth that influences blood clotting and heart disease in later life.

For the moment, lack of nutrition in pregnancy is thought to be the reason for long thin babies and large placentas, which doesn't have to mean that the women who give birth to them are eating poorly. They

DO RIGHT-HANDED PEOPLE
LIVE LONGER THAN LEFT-HANDED PEOPLE?

No, says the U.S. National Institute on Aging, after investigating nearly 4000 people over 65 and recording all deaths in the group over a six-year period. The risk of dying was the same for right- and left-handers. But the life spans of 3000 cricketers listed in *Who's Who of Cricketers* seem to tell a different story. Left-handed bowlers had an average life span of 63.5 years, while right-handers averaged 65.5 years. One theory is that left-handers are more accident prone as they have to use tools designed for right-handers; another is that the tradition of forcing children to be right-handed when they are naturally left-handed distorts the statistics.

could be suffering from anemia or lacking access to certain nutrients. Another suspect could be the state of the father's sperm. Alcohol or mild illness at the time of conception is thought to affect sperm quality. Or the cause may be genetic.

Scientists in Russia are testing the theory of prenatal dietary influences and later heart disease by tracing survivors born before and during the siege of Leningrad, which lasted from 1941 to 1944. The population at the time was severely undernourished, and the health of survivors 50 years later could help confirm or refute the heart disease theory.

New screening techniques could lead to early detection of people at risk. Magnetic resonance imaging (MRI) scans the body and with the aid of a computer can pinpoint areas where there is a potential danger of blocked arteries long before trouble arises. A mobile version, developed in London, can screen people in seconds.

One frightening mystery about heart disease could soon be solved. We all read with fear about apparently fit people who collapse in the middle of a run and die of a heart attack. These individuals usually have normal cholesterol levels and blood pressure, and they're ultra health-conscious too: they exercise, they are not overweight, and they don't drink to excess. What they may have is a genetic defect.

The theory is based on the fact that patients who had suffered a heart attack, but none of the warning signs, were found to carry a gene variant identified as ACE polymorphism (angiotensin-converting enzyme). It gave them a threefold increase in the risk of heart attack compared with people who smoked, had high blood pressure, high cholesterol levels or other conventional risk factors.

Dr. Victor Dzau at Stanford University in California is coordinating research in centers throughout North America and Europe to investigate heart disease treatment. Drugs that act as ACE inhibitors are being used in trials to see if they can slow down the progress of heart disease in patients who have shown symptoms. Already, ACE inhibitors have helped reduce heart failure after coronary thrombosis, and they might one day be part of a protective regime for people at risk through genetic predisposition.

GETTING THE MEASURE OF BLOOD PRESSURE

High blood pressure is a strong predictor of heart disease. Those with the condition who are treated or keep it under control reduce the chance of having a stroke by half, and reduce by 20 percent the chance of developing heart disease. There are no obvious symptoms—headaches and nosebleeds, for instance, bear no relation to blood pressure levels—and the only way to know if yours is normal is to test it. From the age of 50, if you have a family history of heart disease, eat a high-fat diet, smoke or don't exercise, it is a good idea to test your blood pressure every year.

When blood pressure is measured, what you get is the pressure at which the heart pumps blood into the major arteries. When the pressure is too high it overtaxes the heart and blood vessels and can in time damage the kidneys.

Testing gives two figures, one for **systolic pressure**, the highest pressure reached during a heart beat, the other for **diastolic pressure**, the lowest pressure reached during a heart beat. Normal systolic pressure varies with individuals. It can be roughly calculated as 100, plus around 10 years less than the age of the person. Diastolic pressure is considered normal if it is less than 90. For example, for a 30 year old, a healthy average reading is 120 over 80 (also written as 120/80, with the systolic figure usually first). For a 50-year-old man it may be 140 over 90 (140/90). A reading of more than 160/90 in the 50-plus age group is considered on the high side and should be looked into. Anything higher than this would probably merit medical treatment. An older woman's risk of high blood pressure is greater than a man's. A reading over 140/90 for women is considered high. Diastolic readings over 90 in the 60-plus age group probably indicate the need for medical treatment.

Blood pressure usually rises slightly with age as arteries become less elastic. Women and older people generally may suffer from a particular form of raised blood pressure called isolated systolic hypertension (ISH). This means the systolic pressure is raised but the diastolic pressure remains in the normal range. In America, older African American women have twice the rate of ISH as white women or men or African American men. This condition can be controlled by drugs.

Blood pressure varies through the day and according to mood and circumstance. It rises with stress, exercise and smoking, and falls when you are resting or sleeping. It has a habit of rising when it is being tested, and several repeat tests are needed, either with a home kit or at the doctor's office, to get a true reading. Portable systems that take readings throughout the day are available, though even these can artificially raise the readings simply because the users are conscious of them. For borderline readings, it's best to do repeat tests over a period of three to six months.

Consistent borderline readings usually result in standard advice: lose weight; keep alcohol intake to the recommended safe limits; reduce salt intake; stop smoking; exercise more; eat more fiber and less fat; practice relaxation or meditation. High readings are likely to mean going on a lifelong regime of drugs, which in many people do limit the damage.

Some people find they have **blood pressure that's too low**, with readings under 110/60. This is not normally a serious condition, but it can deprive the brain of an adequate supply of blood, which in turn can cause fainting and fatigue. Women are more likely than men to have low blood pressure, and in older people "postural hypotension" as it is called, can cause dizziness and fainting after a sudden movement such as standing up or getting out of bed. Coffee at the end of a meal is said to reduce dizziness, as does getting up slowly. Raising the head of the bed can also help.

ASPIRIN: THE "NEW" WONDER DRUG

Aspirin is becoming known more and more as the wonder drug. Not only does it continue to be the mainstay for arthritis, acting both as painkiller and anti-inflammatory agent, but a study of 300 clinical trials from around the world suggests that almost everyone with a history of heart disease should be taking half an aspirin a day for the rest of their lives. This precaution may also reduce the risk of stroke. Aspirin appears to work for men and (possibly less effectively) for women in middle and old age, and for anyone with high blood pressure. One-half to one tablet a day has also been found to protect against cataract and bowel cancer. One study found that the drug cut by half the number of tiny polyps in the bowel that can lead to cancer of the colon.

Nearly 500 people over a three-year period took half an aspirin daily, and the longer it was taken, the greater the protective effect. Aspirin does have its downside however. It can cause stomach bleeding in some people, and may also cause allergy reactions like skin rashes or tinnitus. Researchers are working on a skin patch which might one day be an acceptable form for some people. Doctors warn against taking aspirin unless there are clear signs of heart disease. As for colon cancer, dietary protection in the form of fiber and fresh fruit and vegetables in many cases will be a safer bet.

Stress has long been associated with high blood pressure and heart disease, on the basis that it produces an abundance of hormones that build up as fatty deposits on the arteries. Some people's arteries may also go into spasm under stressful circumstances. An irregular heartbeat is another reaction. Relaxation and meditation are considered effective and cheap antidotes to stress, and for many years researchers have noted the way patients can control their blood pressure and often reduce medication by using biofeedback machines to alert them to a rise in tension. The machines then monitor responses to relaxation techniques. Relaxation may even reduce blocking in the arteries. You don't need a machine to get the effect. Yoga, relaxation and meditation, in classes or at home with a cassette or instruction book, will also do the trick.

SELF-TESTING KITS

Self-testing kits may be the future way to monitor conditions at home. For now, it is possible to check blood pressure, cholesterol and blood glucose (for diabetics). Readings from blood pressure kits need medical supervision to get an accurate overall interpretation, and cholesterol-test kits have been known to be unreliable.

HEART DISEASE AND WOMEN

At last, medical science is beginning to discriminate in a proper manner and to recognize that "for men, read women too" is just not good enough. The Office of Research on Women's Health was set up by the National Institutes of Health in 1991 to address the inequalities. An article in the *British Medical Journal* in 1993 by Professor of Clinical Gerontology Kay-Tee Khaw states, none too soon, that "We need to know whether the present recommendations for preventing, investigating, and treating coronary heart disease, which are largely based on the experience in white middle-aged men, are equally appropriate in women, elderly patients, and other ethnic groups."

Young women seem to have a built-in protection against heart disease. But once past the menopause, natural or medically induced, the risk of heart disease increases dramatically as the hormone estrogen diminishes. Estrogen is associated with higher levels of HDLs, those substances that help remove cholesterol from the bloodstream.

One in nine women between the ages of 45 and 64 has some form of cardiovascular disease, which includes heart disease, high blood pressure, angina and stroke. After 65, it's one woman in three. Cardiovascular disease is the number-one killer of women aged over 50 in the United States. Women who have heart attacks are twice as likely as men to die within the first few weeks of the attack, and two to three times more likely to suffer a second heart attack within five years of the first.

There are other ways in which diagnosis and treatment should be different for women. Women respond less well to bypass surgery, with a success rate around half that of men, partly because women have smaller blood vessels, which are more difficult to operate on, and partly because women tend to be diagnosed later, when heart disease is more advanced. In around one-third of women presenting classical symptoms, angina turns out to be nonspecific chest pain with no indication of heart disease. (Angina is severe discomfort in the chest, linked to inadequate blood supply to the heart.) Electrocardiogram testing in women gives false positive results in around two-thirds of women, and should be replaced with other testing techniques such as an exercise scanner. Studies on the use of aspirin as a protection against heart disease have been mainly carried out on men; a single study on women showed that it is effective, but less so. Diabetes is a greater risk factor in women, as is increased weight in its own right, independent of other symptoms. And there are the higher levels of cholesterol tolerated by women and blood pressure variations already mentioned.

On top of all this, women are susceptible to **triglycerides**. These are another form of lipid or fat lurking in our bloodstreams. Their carrier is VLDL, the V standing for "very." Too much triglyceride in the blood increases the tendency to form clots. The long-running Framingham Heart Disease Epidemiology Study, which has been monitoring 5000 or so inhabitants of a town in Massachusetts since 1948, has identified triglycerides as an independent risk factor for women. Dr. William Castelli, its director, found that women over 50 in the Framingham population with high triglyceride levels were likely to succumb to heart disease.

The danger level is above 2.3 millimoles per liter, and one way to reduce it is to cut down on sugar and carbohydrates. Another is to add oily fish to the diet. Fish oil capsules have been accepted as a treatment by the British National Health Service to control the condition.

PROTECTION IN HORMONE TREATMENTS

Hormone replacement therapy protects against heart disease in post-menopausal women, in addition to treating hot flashes and reducing the thinning of bones. British and American heart specialists support the use of estrogen replacement for this purpose. The risk of heart attack was reported to be reduced by half when women were given estrogen in a long-term Nurses Health Study though there was no change in the risk of stroke.

How does it work? No one is entirely sure. It could be estrogen's ability to maintain a good balance between HDL and LDL. Or it could be an effect on blood vessels themselves. A small investigation of 11 women with angina, carried out by Dr. Guiseppe Rosano and his team at the UK National Heart and Lung Institute, has produced some clues. The 11 patients had low estrogen levels and were given in turn either estrogen tablets or a placebo (a dummy pill). When taking the estrogen, the women were able to exercise longer and showed better blood supply to the heart muscle than when on the placebo. When exercising, only six experienced chest pains after taking estrogen, compared to all when on the placebo.

Dr. Rosano concluded that estrogen relaxed arteries, which improved blood flow to the heart and reduced the amount of work the heart had to do, particularly during exercise.

MENOPAUSE AND AFTER

Menopause has been described by some eminent doctors as a "deficiency disease," one that only occurs because women live longer than they used to. Nature, they assert, did not intend women to outlive their fertility.

There's another way of looking at this. Older mothers still have to be around to rear their children, especially when they have them late, as they did in the not-so-distant past. Surviving records show that millions of women in the late 19th and early 20th centuries lived long enough to experience a natural menopause. The Office of Population Censuses and Surveys figures for 1901 show that in the UK population, women aged from 45 upward numbered *four million*. By 1931 there were *over seven million* women aged over 45. We know that more people are living longer today, but it is totally untrue to suggest that menopause on a large scale is only a recent phenomenon.

Anthropologist Alan Rogers of the University of Utah suggests that menopause evolved so that a woman maximizes her genetic legacy by being able to concentrate on her lastborn and grandchildren by the time she reaches middle age, rather than wearing herself out by having more and more babies of her own. This at least is a positive view. It is no wonder that women in non-Western cultures seem to take the menopause in their stride and suffer fewer symptoms. Living in a culture that does not have doctors talking about a deficiency disease must help, as does being far away from a pharmaceutical industry that sees the potential in medicalizing menopause.

The age at which most women experience the ceasing of menstrual periods is between 45 and 54. Loss of function of the ovaries and the fall in estrogen levels cause the hormone imbalance that can be followed by a range of symptoms, including hot flashes, night sweats, vaginal dryness, headache, physical aches and pains, tiredness and depression.

Some symptoms of menopause may be as much due to psychological and personal distresses, which could occur at any age, as to hormones. Depression at menopause is, for instance, much more likely to occur in women who already have a long history of this problem. The majority of women don't have depression, mood swings or unexplained fatigue, although many women do experience hot flashes and disturbed sleep, with about one in ten getting them badly. Some, about 5 percent, have vaginal dryness, and even fewer have headaches or aching joints. Symptoms on average last about two years but hot flashes can continue for up to ten. About 25 percent of all women are thought to have severe symptoms.

BONE THINNING OR OSTEOPOROSIS

Everyone, men and women alike, loses bone with age, usually very slowly. In the ten years or so following menopause, one woman in four is said to develop extra-rapid bone loss, which can lead to a painful contraction of the spine and fractures of the forearm, thigh or hip beyond the age of 70. About 300,000 women in the United States suffer a hip fracture every year. Between 12 and 20 percent of them do not survive six months after the fracture, dying of complications such as pneumonia from being bedridden. At least 50 percent of those who do survive suffer a permanent disability, and up to 25 percent need to enter a residential home for long-term care. No wonder doctors see estrogen replacement as a sensible and rational response to a "deficiency disease" caused by lifelong lack of exercise and lack of calcium in the diet combined with low estrogen levels.

OSTEOPOROSIS RISK FACTORS

- Slight build, low weight
- Menopause before the age of 45
- Family history of osteoporosis, especially in close female relatives such as mother or grandmother
- Lack of exercise
- Heavy alcohol intake
- Heavy caffeine intake
- Prolonged bed rest or immobility
- Fair skin
- Lack of sufficient calcium in diet throughout life
- High protein diet, which increases calcium loss
- Vitamin D deficiency, which reduces the body's ability to utilize calcium
- Anorexia
- Smoking. Women who smoke experience a menopause on average three years earlier than those who don't smoke. And if you live with a smoker, but don't smoke yourself, you're at the same

disadvantage. The earlier the menopause, the longer the risk of thinning bones.

- Early hysterectomy. Removal of the uterus and ovaries brings on an early menopause and an earlier start to bone loss. Even when the ovaries are not removed, they cease to function in the majority of women within two to four years after hysterectomy.

- Long-term use of steroids. Taken regularly as a treatment for arthritis or to prevent asthma, steroids can lead to bone loss. There's no way of predicting who will or will not lose bone through taking steroids regularly.

THE CALCIUM CONNECTION

Extra calcium in the diet is needed after the menopause (see Chapter Two) on ways to get it. A publication from the National Institute on Aging, called simply *Menopause*, explains clearly the connection between hormones and calcium: "Estrogen helps bones absorb the calcium they need to stay strong. It also helps conserve the calcium stored in the bones by encouraging other cells to use dietary calcium more efficiently. For instance, muscles require calcium to contract. If there is not enough calcium circulating in the blood for muscles to use, calcium is 'borrowed' from the bone. Calcium is also needed for blood clotting, sending nerve impulses, and secreting various hormones. Prolonged borrowing from bone calcium for these processes speeds bone loss."

You are less at risk if . . .

. . . you have ever been pregnant. Reasons: increased intake of calcium-rich foods, which many pregnant women include in their diet; high levels of estrogen during pregnancy boost vitamin D productivity, which in turn promotes calcium absorption; the hormone progesterone, present in higher levels in pregnancy, adds to the bone-conserving effect.

. . . you have taken the contraceptive pill. There's some evidence that women who have taken oral contraceptives for a long time have denser bones than women who have not; the hormones in oral contraceptives

may stimulate release of a substance called calcitonin, which inhibits bone breakdown.

. . . *you are slightly overweight.* Greater body weight puts more stress on the bones, just as exercise does. And, after menopause, where there's fat there's also the chance to store more estrogen—in the fat cells.

. . . *you have the right genes.* Women whose mothers did not suffer from osteoporosis are also less likely to do so; studies show that black people have stronger, thicker, larger bones than does the white population. Black women tend to lose bone more slowly than white women, and lose less calcium in their urine. Black and white men, however, lose bone and calcium in similar amounts.

DOES SCREENING MAKE SENSE?

The screening techniques developed in recent years can measure bone density to some extent, but they are not very accurate in their readings and they do not predict which women will go on to have a fracture in later years. Only about a third of women found to have low bone density through screening are likely to experience later fractures. The Leeds University School of Public Health study investigated the value of screening and estimated that a national program in the United Kingdom would lead to the prevention of only 5 percent of the fractures suffered by elderly women. Adding this to the lack of knowledge about the long-term effect of hormone replacement, the team concluded that "other strategies" would be more appropriate, including diet advice, exercise, giving up smoking and promoting safety in the homes of older people.

It is likely that a gene for osteoporosis will be found, and an accurate way of screening will follow. Already, researchers at Thomas Jefferson University in Philadelphia have found a defect in a gene for a type of collagen in a patient with osteoporosis.

Current screening methods can be useful for those in a high-risk category. Even if hormone replacement is not used, there is the value of a timely warning that could lead the way to a healthier lifestyle. The screening machines are called densitometers. They also expose bones to small doses of radiation, considered to be well within safety limits. Results usually show up in minutes on a computer screen. As a rough guide, the quicker the readout, the lower the dose of radiation. One new machine uses ultrasound instead, and measures the heel bone. All current versions of scanning share a problem: There is no automatic relationship between the state of bones in different parts of the body. For instance, losing bone in the wrist does not necessarily indicate bone loss in the hip.

HORMONE REPLACEMENT THERAPY

Osteoporosis is the main reason doctors today take such a keen interest in estrogen replacement. Hormone replacement can effectively reduce or eliminate the symptoms of menopause by restoring levels of estrogen. The hormone is given alone ("unopposed") to women who have had a hysterectomy, in which case it may be called estrogen replacement therapy (ERT). However, for those with an intact uterus, estrogen alone has in the past led to endometrial cancer, cancer of the lining of the uterus. The hormone progestin (a synthetic version of progesterone) protects against this, but produces monthly break-through bleeding. The combined treatment is often called Hormone Replacement Therapy (HRT).

The HRT story sounds like nothing less than total success. Women can preserve their bones, avoid temporary menopausal symptoms and protect themselves against heart disease. There's even evidence to suggest that HRT preserves muscle strength, and this contributes to prevention of bone breakage.

But all is not straightforward. HRT, begun in the years first following menopause, will protect bone, but medical opinion differs over whether it will rebuild it. A study published in 1993, in the *New England Journal of Medicine*, concluded that HRT preserved bone only when taken for at least seven to nine years, a commitment inviting some risk (see below). The study also showed that as soon as the women stopped taking HRT their bone density declined rapidly. By the age of 75, their levels were only slightly higher than in women who had never used hormone replacement.

The doctors working on this study maintained that HRT increased bone density as well as preserving it, and they recommend that the treatment can be started at the age of 70 and will still reduce risk of fracture by a third. But at the present time, there simply have not been enough women taking HRT for the number of years needed to assess safety or effectiveness. Only about 15 percent of women eligible for hormone replacement are now receiving it in the United States. Most of these will have stopped within a couple of years, either because their menopausal symptoms have declined, or because they did not wish to put up with side effects, or because they disliked the idea of being on a treatment for life.

HOW MUCH, HOW LONG ON HORMONE REPLACEMENT?

For menopausal symptoms, normally one to five years. For bone protection, at least ten years and probably for life.

The risks: up to five years seems to be safe; between five and ten years is a gray area needing further monitoring; over ten years the risk of breast cancer increases by 30 percent. Putting it another way, the incidence of breast cancer rises from ten women per 10,000 to 13 women per 10,000 a year. *Anyone on hormone replacement needs regular breast screening, once or twice a year.*

Who shouldn't take hormone replacement? Anyone with a history of breast cancer, a tendency to blood clotting, severe varicose veins, gall bladder disease or endometriosis. Also acute liver disease, pancreatic disease or stroke. Doctors are divided about giving estrogen replacement to

---

DOES HORMONE REPLACEMENT THERAPY REJUVENATE?

Clearer skin, better hair textures, more energy and increased libido have all been reported in women using hormone replacement. It's not all in the mind either. Estrogen does thicken skin and improve hair growth, and if the vasoconstriction associated with migraine and headache is reduced, it's not surprising that spirits rise. But fluid retention is a common side effect of hormone replacement therapy, and the combined version containing progesterone is connected with depression. Win some, lose some.

women with high blood pressure, benign breast disease, migraine or epilepsy, or to cigarette smokers.

Any side effects? Progestins can cause bloating, breast tenderness, headaches, depression and irregular bleeding. Estrogen can cause nausea, leg cramps and breast tenderness. A small gain in weight is not uncommon.

Ways to take the hormones: In tablet form, either every day or over a three-week cycle; in the form of a patch stuck to the abdomen or thigh, which is replaced either every few days or weekly; as a vaginal cream purely to relieve vaginal dryness over the short term.

Disadvantages: All methods cause breakthrough bleeding when combined hormones are taken, though newer compounds may avoid this. Patches can cause local skin irritation. Vaginal creams are only for vaginal dryness and can be absorbed by a partner and do not provide a sufficient dose to protect against osteoporosis or heart disease.

OTHER BONE PRESERVERS AND MAKERS

Biphosphonates are a group of drugs that reduce bone deterioration and restore small amounts of bone. The kind used for osteoporosis is called elindxonate disodium (trade name Fosamax). It is suitable for women and men with diagnosed osteoporosis who may have suffered fractures, and is taken in tablet form alternating with calcium supplements, sometimes in addition to HRT. Vitamin D supplements might be added. The treatment is prescribed for a period of three years. Didronel has been described for osteoporosis for only six years, but the drug has a ten-year safety record in treating Paget's disease, another bone condition. It is not suitable for people with a history of kidney problems or colitis.

Calcitonin is produced naturally by the thyroid gland to maintain levels of calcium and other minerals. Production declines with age and the lower levels could contribute to osteoporosis. A form of calcitonin derived from salmon has been found to preserve bone and restore small amounts if taken for a year. Calcitonin, combined with calcium, may be used to help people diagnosed as having osteoporosis. It is given by injection or in a nasal spray form.

Fluoride can increase bone density, though it can also, in high amounts, increase the risk of hip fractures, and there is a theory that it produces low-quality bone replacement. It has been given to patients with very severe osteoporosis of the spine, sometimes combined with calcitonin and/or calcium. The side effects may not be acceptable—gastrointestinal bleeding, leg pains and nausea.

Ipriflavone, a preparation based on an organic extract from plants, promises a new, non-hormonal approach in the prevention and treatment of osteoporosis. This one could mean that women who cannot take HRT will be offered a viable alternative.

THE MALE MENOPAUSE?

If hormone replacement does something for women, could it do anything for men? The answer, a little tentatively, is yes. The GH, or growth hormone, factor and its rejuvenating effects are described on page 79, and is clearly nowhere near safe enough on a long-term basis. But the male hormone testosterone, an equivalent to the female hormone estrogen, declines gradually from about the age of 60 or 65, and supplements may strengthen muscles and reduce frailty in elderly men, though its effectiveness has not been proved. A precursor of this hormone DHEA (for deyhydroepiandrosterone) is also being looked at for its positive effects on the immune system and protection against chronic disease.

Testosterone replacement therapy (TRT) has been used successfully on a small scale for some years by British doctor Malcolm Carruthers, head of the Hormonal Healthcare Centre in London. He treats for what he refers to as the "male menopause," a dramatic fall in testosterone levels that occurs in a minority of men according to current knowledge, and he claims that testosterone therapy can improve skin texture, increase energy and libido, protect against thinning bone and act as an anti-stress agent against heart disease.

Now Dr. Carruthers is shifting his attention to a protein that makes the body testosterone-resistant, called SHBG (for sex hormone binding globulin), a substance that increases with age. He's giving testosterone supplements to reverse the effect, though his patients also need to cut out smoking, reduce drinking, lose weight and avoid stress. Testosterone supplements can increase the risk of prostate cancer and the medical profession has yet to be convinced of the value of Dr. Carruthers' work. Meanwhile, he is planning his own clinics in the United States, using European-produced testosterone which he claims is safer than the United States variety.

COLD BATHS

Cold baths can improve the immune system and extend life, says Professor Vijay Kakkar of the Thrombosis Research Institute in London. Professor Kakkar claims positive results with patients suffering from chronic fatigue syndrome after persuading sufferers to take a daily 20-minute cold-water bath. Weakness and exhaustion just disappeared.

He says the treatment also boosts sexual potency and regulates fertility by enhancing production of the male hormone testosterone and the female hormone estrogen. And it thins the blood, which could reduce the risk of blood clotting. It has also cured Professor Kakkar's asthma.

In case you can't wait to rush into a cold bath, there is a little more to it than one might think. Thermo-Regulatory Hydrotherapy (TRHT), to give the proper name, involves four stages of adaptation, building up to the heroic 20 minutes and a gradual lowering of the temperature to 60 degrees Farenheit. Not for those with heart disease or other chronic illnesses.

Professor Kakkar, a respected surgeon, was so anxious to pass on his regime that he published his findings in a special edition of *The European* newspaper rather than wait for the cumbersome processes of medical journals—although they are on the agenda along with further trials. TRHT involves no drugs and has been used since the 19th century in European spas. All Professor Kakkar is adding are some scientific theories, such as the idea that the effect may be partly due to an increase in white blood cells, affecting immune-system functioning. Others are watching his research with cautious interest.

ALZHEIMER'S—
A DISEASE STILL LOOKING FOR A CURE

In 1907 a German doctor, Alois Alzheimer, used a new technique in a postmortem on a 51-year-old woman who had suffered memory loss and personality changes in the last few years of her life. He found that her brain contained dark spots, which he rightly assumed to be connected to her condition. These spots are now known as neurofibrillary tangles and senile plaques, caused by a substance called beta amyloid which deposits itself in the brain of sufferers. They result in interference with transmission of brain signals and chemicals in brain cells.

Alzheimer's is a major disease in the Western world. It currently affects four million Americans, mainly over 65. The disease can also strike those as young as 40. Between the ages of 65 and 74 the estimated incidence is 1 person in 25; at 85 and over, the incidence is at least 1 in 5.

The symptoms for Alzheimer's disease vary with individuals. Often it looks like mere forgetfulness or even depression at first. Sometimes there seems to be erratic or eccentric behavior. The disease tends to be spotted when there are continued signs of forgetfulness or confusion, such as going out shopping and then forgetting the purpose of the excursion, or making a meal and either forgetting to eat it or immediately thinking it is necessary to make another meal because the first has slipped from the memory. Leaving ovens or tea kettles on or continually losing items are other possible signs. And loss of smell is suspected of being an early indicator—Alzheimer's sufferers need extra concentration to identify odors.

A certain amount of memory loss is normal with age, but Alzheimer's is not a normal part of the aging process and it is a mystery as to why some people develop the condition. One new way of thinking is that there is a whole family of Alzheimer's diseases, some with early and some with late onset. Head injury may be a cause, drinking water containing aluminum is also suspected. In comparatively rare cases, there's a family history. The consensus is that there is a host of genetic errors, with many different triggers for the destructive amyloid effect.

IS ALUMINUM DANGEROUS?

Fears that aluminum could be a cause of Alzheimer's disease tend to be dismissed by many medical experts who say the case is unproven. Professor Derek Birchall of Keele University points out that only a trace of aluminum is absorbed from water, foil and other common agents and even then the amount varies in individuals. Even so, in areas where levels of aluminum in the water supply are high, there is a 50 percent increase in the number of cases, and at least six separate studies link the disease to aluminum. It could be prudent to cut down on use of aluminum cooking pots and aluminum-containing antacids. Professor Birchall also suggests adding the mineral silicon to water supplies high in aluminum after finding that it reduces absorption by 85 percent. Silicon tablets could be equally protective.

TESTS AND TREATMENTS

At the National Institutes of Health, Dr. Daniel Alkon is working on blood and skin tests that measure potassium function and could lead to a way of diagnosing Alzheimer's disease. Not all dementia is caused by Alzheimer's. Stroke or possibly hardening of the arteries, both of which interrupt blood flow to the brain, could trigger similar symptoms. About 50 percent of cases of dementia, or loss of mental function, are due to other conditions that may well be treatable. A gene for Alzheimer's called Apoe-4 was identified in 1993, and this could lead to screening the general population in the not-too-distant future, with the promise of 90 percent accuracy. This prospect fills many scientists with doom and gloom, since there are no cures, and the promise could seem more like a death sentence to someone in middle age or younger who receives bad news.

No cures, maybe, but already there are treatments that slow the progress of the disease and temporarily limit brain cell damage. Tacrine is thought to prevent the breakdown of a certain chemical transmitter in the brain called acetylcholine. It reverses symptoms or stops them from worsening for a time, though after about four years the positive effect wears off. A protein called Nerve Growth Factor may stimulate the growth of nerve cells in Alzheimer's patients and could lead to another effective drug.

There is a cluster of new so-called "smart drugs," notably centrophenoxine, deprenyl, hydergine, piracetum and phosphatidylserine, which have been seen to enhance memory concentration and communication skills for a short time in some sufferers. But the positive effect is not consistent and the findings are based on a small body of research in humans.

CHECKS ON CANCER

Gene therapy promises to change the way many cancers will be treated in the next ten years. But for the moment, much of the emphasis is on prevention and screening. In the United States, deaths from stomach cancer have fallen 85 percent since the 1930s, and this is attributed to including more fresh foods in the diet. The newer free radical theories and dietary guidelines, and awareness of smoking dangers, should change the picture even more. Even so, there have been increases in non-smoking related cancer deaths in people over 55.

Screening has proved its value with many cancers. Here is a list of tests available that could lead to early treatment and often cure.

BREAST CANCER

Mammogram x-rays can pick up a potential problem up to two years before a lump is felt. Screening before the menopause is a controversial topic. It's not reliable, the radiation dose could be harmful and survival rates do not merit wide-scale screening, say some doctors. Others claim increased survival rates in younger age groups taking part in screening programs.

Opinions vary on screening older women too. The American Cancer Society has recommended a baseline mammogram by the age of 40, followed by screening mammograms every one or two years, then yearly after the age of 50. British specialists suggest that any doctor offering mammograms to women under 50 should also issue warnings of possible radiation risk. Monthly self-checks for breast lumps are advised for women of all ages, along with a yearly professional breast exam.

Tamoxifen, a nonsteroid anti-estrogen hormone used to prevent recurrence of breast cancer, has been on trial at London's Royal Marsden's Hospital as a protection which might be offered to women with a family history of breast cancer. Volunteers who have never suffered from breast cancer themselves, but have a family history of the disease, have been taking the hormone. Tamoxifen can reduce cholesterol levels and bone loss, but its future as a preventive in women who have never had breast cancer may be limited, as the research is beginning to show that it may itself trigger other kinds of cancer.

Some recent research questions the link between breast cancer and a family history of the disease, but the conventional view is that the risk is one in six for women whose mothers were diagnosed over the age of 50, and one in four if their mother was diagnosed when she was under 50. If the maternal grandmother and other close female relatives have been affected, the risk is again increased. The risk without a family history is one in 12.

The incidence of breast cancer is linked to the length of a woman's reproductive life, with a higher risk associated with early menstruation and later menopause. The vitamin-rich antioxidant diet may offer protection, as described in Chapter 2. Large studies in the United States and the Netherlands have disproved the link between fatty foods and breast cancer.

CERVICAL CANCER

A pelvic examination and Pap smear test are advised every year for older women, though after three normal results in women over 65, screening can be dropped for one to three years.

The Pap smear test has come under criticism for giving inaccurate results due to laboratory errors, and a new test has been developed in

Australia that uses a computer-aided probe and promises to be speedy and accurate.

COLON CANCER

Colon, or bowel, cancer increases with age and is one of the most common cancers, but caught early the survival rate is quite high. There are three tests: a rectal examination; a "fecal occult" test that can detect unseen blood in stool samples; and a sigmoidoscopy, a rectal examination involving a flexible scope. The first two are advised as part of a yearly check-up for women and men over 50, and the latter is recommended at age 50 and then every three to five years.

In the United Kingdom, trial screening tests point to the usefulness of sigmoidoscopy every three to five years in people who have a family history of bowel, breast, endometrial or ovarian cancer, or who have longstanding and extensive colitis. Anyone with rectal bleeding, a change in regular bowel habits or ano-rectal pain would be candidates for the test, too. Often these conditions have no connection with colon cancer, but if the cause is a precancerous polyp in the rectum, it can be easily removed if found early.

The fecal occult test has not been proved as reliable in detecting cancer. However, a trial of nearly 50,000 volunteers, submitting annual feces samples for examination (on strips of chemically impregnated paper) showed up many symptomless colon cancers at a curable stage. The volunteers were followed up for 13 years, and when compared to others tested once in two years or not at all, there were a third fewer deaths from colon cancer.

PROSTATE CANCER

More than 80 percent of prostate cancer cases occur in men aged 65 and over, but it can happen in men as young as 45. The American Cancer Society recommends that men 50 and older have a yearly PSA (Prostate-specific antigen) test, backed up if necessary by further tests. A procedure launched in 1994 examines density of new blood vessels in the prostate and can predict with greater accuracy the progression of a tumor from early signs, meaning in some cases that only minor treatment or monitoring (watchful waiting) is needed.

SKIN CANCER

A vaccine against skin cancer is the great hope among researchers worldwide. Trials are already showing encouraging results, with many more patients given a vaccine remaining tumor-free after treatments compared to those not vaccinated. A gene protecting against skin cancer has been identified by doctors in the United Kingdom funded by the Imperial Cancer Research Fund. Those lucky enough to be born with it have a built-in protection against skin cancer, and the finding could lead to a cure. In the meantime, the usual checks on changes in warts and moles still hold true.

Even if you have kept out of the sun for years, a lifetime of exposure can result in a mole changing size, shape or color, or inflammation, itching, oozing or bleeding in later life. Many of these changes individually do not mean skin cancer, but a combination could, and early detection can mean cure. Get medical advice if you notice any changes in a mole or other skin changes.

OVARIAN CANCER

Early detection of ovarian cancer can save lives. The survival rate is almost 90 percent if the condition is detected before it has time to spread. Unfortunately, it can remain symptomless until too late. A Pap test does not screen for ovarian cancer. New screening techniques undergoing trial under Dr. Ian Jacobs of the Royal London Hospital use a blood test and ultrasound and could lead the way to new kinds of screening, especially for women with a family history of ovarian cancer.

SELF-EXAMS

Testicular self-exam, done once a month in a warm bath or shower, could mean early detection and cure. Rest the scrotum in the palms of your hands and use the thumb and fingers of both hands to examine each of the testicles in turn. Don't worry about slight differences in size, which is normal. Check for lumps, swellings and any marked difference in weight. You will feel the epididymis, a tube that transports sperm, at the top and back of the testicle.

Breast self-exams once a month are proven as an early detector of breast lumps. Stand in front of a mirror in good light and look first at the general shape of your breasts, checking for any change in appearance such as skin puckering or difference in shape. Raise each arm in turn and again check appearance, then raise both arms and check both sides in profile. Examine your right breast lying on your back with your right hand supporting your head. Use the three middle fingers of your left hand to feel in a circular movement around the breast. Press gently and in the same circular motion check up to your armpit and collarbone for any lumps and swellings there.

Repeat with the left breast. Then take each quarter of breast, moving fingers inward to nipple, feeling for any changes. Repeat on the other side.

HEALTH CARE AS WE AGE

Serious and life-threatening diseases are not a normal part of healthy aging. It's the smaller ailments, the result of wear and tear, that bother most of us.

Symptoms that we've learned to live with, that have come and gone for years—such as mild indigestion, the odd headache and general aches and pains—are no reason for worry. Symptoms that slowly get worse—*more* headaches, persistent tiredness or whatever—are worth a visit to the doctor. You could find you have migraine, or an underactive thyroid or arthritis or some other condition that is not self-limiting and could be treated. Symptoms that are *new* and continue for a week or two, gradually getting worse, also need attention.

Aging affects the way our bodies metabolize drugs, almost always adversely. We eliminate drugs from our bodies more slowly, so there are higher amounts present in the body for longer periods. This is partly due to slower metabolism and reduction in liver size and blood flow.

And we become more sensitive to drugs, experiencing more adverse reactions. Up to 25 percent of elderly patients admitted to the hospital experience adverse drug reactions says Ken Woodhouse, Professor of Geriatric Medicine at the University of Wales College of Medicine. The older we get, the more likely we are to be prescribed drugs by our doctors. There is an urgent need for more research into this field, so that the dose is better tailored to meet the needs of older patients.

AGEISM AND ILLNESS

Are older people subjected to adverse discrimination by the medical profession? Is the category "geriatric" an excuse for stereotyping and should it therefore be abolished? As the population of Western countries ages, we are in danger of seeing older people denied treatment in the name of "priorities" and on the basis of their lower life expectancy. There is a danger that economic policies will prevent medical advances from reaching older populations. Current examples are not encouraging.

If you are over 65, live in the United Kingdom and want a flu vaccine, make sure your doctor is over 50. When asked to whom they'd offer the vaccination, only one-third of doctors aged under 35 said they'd consider it for all of their patients over 65, while over half of doctors aged over 50 did so. A survey of those in charge of coronary care in the United Kingdom revealed that an age-related admissions policy was being ob-

THE IMPORTANCE OF IMMUNIZATION

Immunization can reduce the death rate from influenza by 50 percent or more among those in older age groups. One-third of people over 60 catching flu and three-quarters over 70 are likely to develop bronchitis. In the United States, many doctors recommend that the following people have an annual vaccination: adults over age 65; adults with chronic heart, lung or kidney disease; adults with diabetes or an immune disorder; and nursing home residents. Vaccination also makes sense for anyone who has asthma or is on steroids.

served, with limits ranging from age 65 to 80. Clot-busting drugs, which can make a marked difference in survival after a heart attack, were in use in only 9 percent of geriatric wards. In the United States too, a 75-year-old is only half as likely to receive these drugs as is a 40-year-old, though they are more useful for older than younger patients.

The prejudices of the medical profession are something we must, as we age, be aware of and resist. How do we do it?

If you are in doubt or dissatisfied, get a second opinion. Except for emergency surgery, always ask the doctor to explain what is the matter with you. Bear the following in mind and try to drum up the courage to ask:

- Has the diagnosis been confirmed by all necessary tests?
- What are the appropriate treatments?
- Do treatments have side effects or risks?
- If surgery is recommended, what are the benefits?
- If surgery is normally advised, but not in this case, why not?
- What are the consequences if I don't want surgery, and if I do?
- How familiar is the surgeon with the particular operation? (The more often a surgeon performs it, the more competent he or she will be.)
- If costs are involved, what will they be, and are all contingencies covered?

BUNDLE UP

Many more older people die in winter than in summer, a phenomenon that has been put down to hypothermia, or body chilling through lack of heat, despite the fact that modern heating and house insulation should have greatly reduced the risk. Now doctors are beginning to suspect that the chilling happens out of doors through wearing too-flimsy clothing when waiting for a bus, watching football or other low-effort activities. Prolonged chilling can lead to pneumonia, strokes and heart attack. The best protection for going out in the cold is warm, layered clothing, plus a hat. About 80 percent of body heat loss can be through an unprotected head.

BODY MAINTENANCE—
THE PARTS THAT DON'T HAVE TO WEAR OUT

Sight, hearing, teeth, feet, joints, lungs and bladder all show the wear and tear of time. Here are a few pointers for taking care of the body and knowing when to get professional help.

EYESIGHT

One of the earliest reminders of aging is the need to wear reading glasses, a development occurring from around the mid-40s in people who previously had normal vision. In warmer climates, this happens in the 30s for reasons that remain a mystery. Decline in visual acuity is a result of the eyes' lenses losing their flexibility; there's no cure, though surgery to implant lenses for close vision is currently being tested in the United States.

Color perception changes with age, with the lens of the eye of a 40-year-old transmitting, for example, 30 percent of the blue light of the sky compared to 2 to 3 percent at the age of 80. This means we may be choosing brighter colors than we think for our clothes or decor as we age, and should be a little vigilant if our natural inclination is toward muted shades. We also become more sensitive to glare, which can be a nuisance when driving at night. Some people benefit from special anti-glare glasses for night driving.

Bright sunshine and ultraviolet light produce a haze over older eyes known as fluorescence. A peaked hat or yellowish sunglasses reduce the haze, which is no doubt why, without even being told, many elderly people favor caps and other headgear.

KEEPING YOUR EYES FROM STRAIN

- Lighting is important at any age, but normal healthy eyes at the age of 40 need twice as much illumination as they do at 20, and three times as much at 60. Use an adjustable light for close work.

- VDT screens can be hard on the eyes. Take 10- to 15-minute breaks every hour, blink often to lubricate your eyes, and every now and then look away from close work into the distance, or even stare at a blank wall.

- Soothe tired eyes with cool, damp teabags or a slice of cucumber on each closed eye. Leave them in place and relax for ten minutes. Or try this "palming" exercise: Sit up straight, removing glasses. Rest your elbows on the table and keep your back straight. Place palms over eyeballs, resting the heel of your hands on cheekbones, with fingers crossing over each other on your forehead. Then visualize something soothing and calming like the sea or a mountain against a blue sky, concentrating for up to five minutes.

- Spots and specks that float across the field of vision are usually normal and harmless. If the spots change suddenly or they are accompanied by flashing lights, get your eyes checked.

- Dry eyes can result in itching or reduced vision, and need a check. Special eyedrop solutions can usually correct the problem. A reduction in tear flow is normal with age, but the dryness is not.

- Excessive watering is usually nothing more than increased sensitivity to light, wind and temperature change. Sunglasses with protective lenses will often solve the problem. Excessive watering can be due to loss of elasticity in the lower eyelid. Wipe your eyes sideways, not down, to avoid stretching delicate tissue. If watering is excessive, it could be a sign of a blocked tear duct or eye infection.

- Cataracts are cloudy areas of the eye which obscure vision. They are common in people aged over 70, and can lead to blindness. Modern surgery, often requiring only a local anesthetic, can correct the problem in at least 90 percent of cases.

- What you eat may determine whether or not you develop cataracts—and again it's those antioxidants that count. Studies have demonstrated a low intake of vitamin C and beta-carotene in cataract patients. Other protective nutrients noted in studies are B$_2$ (riboflavin), vitamin A, zinc oxide, vitamin E and selenium. Aspirin may also offer protection, a phenomenon noticed in arthritis sufferers who take aspirin as a painkiller and do not develop cataracts.

- Diarrhea and cataracts are linked, especially in developing countries. The reason seems to be that the kidneys become less efficient at removing the harmful waste products of digestion, and the toxins build up and damage the eye.

- Glaucoma occurs when there is too much fluid pressure in the eye, which can in time destroy vision. Long-term steroid treatment increases the risk of the condition. Early diagnosis and treatment can control symptoms, but regular eye pressure checks from the age of 40 for anyone with a family history of glaucoma are needed as there's usually no pain or other symptoms at the outset.

- Age-related macular degeneration is one of the most common causes of blindness in the Western world. The macula is the part of the retina responsible for sharp focusing, and it can stop functioning efficiently with age. Signs are blurring of reading vision and deterioration of the central part of vision but not side or peripheral vision. Laser treatment may help if the condition is detected early. Vitamin supplements could halt or prevent deterioration, according to some studies.

Screening every two years is advisable from about the age of 45 on in order to pick up serious eye problems early and check that glasses correction is still correct.

HEARING

The ability to hear clearly begins to decline at the comparatively early age of 30. High-pitched sounds are the first to go. Gradually, differentiation between sounds becomes impaired, which is why it gets harder and harder to follow a conversation in a noisy restaurant or crowded party. Around one-third of people over 65 experience serious hearing loss. Many do not seek help either because they don't wish to admit a handicap or they don't realize that their hearing is sufficiently damaged to merit medical attention.

How hearing can be helped:

- Go to your doctor for a checkup if any of these begin to happen: You find it hard to follow a conversation; you have to turn up the television or radio so loud that the family complains; you find yourself asking people to repeat things; you often miss hearing the doorbell or telephone.

- Wax in the ear could be the easily solved problem. Wax becomes harder as we age and less likely to clear on its own. It can accumulate into a hard plug and impair hearing. You can buy over-the-counter remedies that may soften and dissolve the wax, though you may still have to see your doctor to arrange for syringing afterward. As a preventive, every six months put a few drops of olive oil into the ear, morning and night for three to five days, with a wad of cotton wool to stop seepage.

- Hearing aids take some getting used to, but they do work fairly well when used in conversation with one or two people. Modern technology still hasn't found a way to get them to operate well against background noise, and that goes for costly and inexpensive devices alike.

- With or without a hearing aid, make it easier for yourself by choosing restaurants with carpets and draperies and preferably no background music. Soft surfaces absorb noise better than hard ones.

- Tinnitus, persistent ringing or other noise in ears, affects about 20 percent of those over 65. Mostly, it is due to degenerative changes in the middle or inner ear, but sometimes the cause is an allergy—not uncommon in those taking aspirin—or it could be stress. Not an easy one to overcome. A masker producing "white noise" may help some people.

- Can lost hearing ever be regained? Retinoic acid, the vitamin A derivative used to rejuvenate aging skin, has been reported as reinstating hearing in rats. This research could lead to help for humans, too.

TEETH

It is an unfortunate fact of life that tooth decay isn't just for kids. We can go on getting cavities as long as we have our own teeth. Adults are more vulnerable to root cavities, in the space where the gums have receded through periodontal disease. The trouble can begin from about the age of 35. Receding gums expose a portion of the tooth that is not coated with protective enamel. The teeth become loose in time, and the whole process leads ultimately to tooth extraction.

Ways to retain your own teeth:

- Floss, brush and have twice-a-year checkups—these are the rules for preventive dental care.

- Brush twice a day, *for at least three minutes each session.* Count each brush stroke per second or use a timer. Brushing itself is more important than toothpaste as a way to remove decay-causing food and plaque (the sticky mucous coating that contains bacteria and leads to cavities).

- Floss daily for debris between the teeth, and always carry a supply of toothpicks to use, with care, after meals if needed.

- For tender, bleeding gums, try a mouthwash or simply rinse with a tumbler of warm water with a teaspoon of salt added.

- Toothpastes usually have an abrasive action for attacking bacteria. The ideal kind should contain an antiplaque formula. Toothpastes labeled "natural" are less likely to contain harsh chemicals or artificial colors and sweeteners and may have such ingredients as fennel, which acts as a natural antibacterial agent, or propolis, which is claimed to be a gum stimulant.

- Whiteners often contain peroxide, which is not good for the enamel. Check on the label before buying.

- Gum disease affects about 95 percent of adults and is due to a buildup of plaque around the gum line. Inflammation of the gums can lead to loosened teeth and bone loss.

- Tartar is the hard deposit on teeth that hygienists have to scrape off. It is caused by plaque and minerals in the saliva and does little harm as long as it is cleaned off regularly.

- At menopause and after, some women experience a dry mouth or a burning mouth sensation, which estrogen therapy may alleviate for reasons unknown. Giving up spicy foods for a while may also help.

- Sensitivity to hot and cold is caused by receding gums, which expose dentine, the layer under the tooth enamel. Toothpastes for sensitive gums usually take about two weeks before they coat or desensitize the dentine. Best to use them from time to time as needed.

- Though fluoride in the water supply is considered the best and cheapest way to reduce tooth decay, some people object to the idea and there are claims of side effects such as bone-weakening. However, the medical establishment accepts the value of fluoride to protect adult as well as youthful teeth, and fluoride toothpastes and mouth rinses for daily or weekly use may be useful.

FEET

Just over 50 percent of people aged 75 to 79 could cut their own toenails in a survey by podiatrists of 536 patients aged 75 and over. Only 23 percent at 90-plus could do so. Men did better than women, but then men generally have fewer foot problems than women, which is thought to reflect the fact that men wear more sensible shoes. The most common trouble in the survey was hallux valgus, a deformed big toe, which distorts the joint and is due to wearing too-small shoes. Hammertoe, the result of shortening of the tendons that control toe movement, was also common. In severe cases, surgery may be recommended. Avoid this by wearing well-fitting shoes. Very few in the survey said their mobility was hindered, which is something to be cheerful about.

Feet may gradually change shape with age, especially through added weight. Just because you had a slim foot shape in youth, don't assume

LEG ULCERS

Many more older women than men get leg ulcers, and though they may heal, thin skin means even a very minor injury can open the wound again. Potential sufferers could be detected in their 40s or 50s by using ultrasound, which would show up leaky valves in the vascular system, but at present there are no plans for such screening.

that you still have it. Problems can develop through neglect—it's all too easy to take feet for granted, bullying them into too-tight shoes, letting them slip about in too-loose ones, ignoring minor discomforts until they becomes major ones. Corns, for instance, are caused by friction and pressure on bony areas of the foot caused by rubbing against shoes.

How to keep feet fit:

- Start with well-fitting footwear, with uppers made of soft but supportive leather. High heels are best kept for special occasions, preferably when there won't be too much standing. Make sure shoes are wide enough across and long enough at the toes—there should be a half-inch gap between the ends of your toes and the ends of your shoes, and a snug fit at heel and instep. You get the best support with laces or straps.

- Buy shoes in the afternoons when your feet are likely to be a little swollen. Walk around the shop to make sure toes don't come to the end of the shoe when you're standing.

- Slippers are sloppy and most of them give little support. Ditto with espadrilles and other soft fabric shoes. Wear them sparingly to avoid the muscle strain that can lead to spurs or the calcium growths that can develop on the bones of the foot.

- Change socks and stockings every day to keep fungal and bacterial conditions at bay. They occur because feet provide them an ideal dark, damp, warm environment. Wash and dry feet thoroughly, using a fungicidal powder if you are prone to infection.

- Don't go for tight garters or too-tight socks that can restrict circulation.

- Dry skin can lead to itching and burning. Massage feet with a body moisturizer after washing.

- Over-the-counter remedies can sometimes alleviate calluses, corns and warts, using acids that burn off the tissue or support pads that reduce the pressure. If the problem recurs or is very painful, professional help is needed.

- Anyone suffering from diabetes or circulation problems needs to discuss foot ailments with a doctor before trying any do-it-yourself cures.

- Do your heels ache when you wake in the morning? It's almost certainly from pressure caused by heavy bed covers. Try placing a rolled pillow at the bottom of the bed under the covers to lift them higher than your feet.

- Ingrown toenails are a result of cutting the toenails incorrectly. Cut straight across, never in a curve around the nail, and keep the nails longer than the sides of the nail bed.

- Keep feet supple with stretch and strengthening exercises. Do these daily:

  1. Stand with feet parallel and rise on tiptoes, going up and down four times.

  2. Sit down and stretch one foot and leg straight in front, first pointing the toes and then extending the instep. Stretch, then relax; repeat four times for each foot.

  3. Still sitting, extend one foot at a time and rotate from the ankle in circles, four circles each way.

ARE ATHLETIC SHOES GOOD FOR OLDER FEET?

There are two views on this. Researchers at Bristol University recommended athletic shoes for arthritis sufferers to reduce the impact on painful joints when walking. The well-padded heels of athletic shoes act as a shock absorber. But thickness in the sole of shoes is also associated with instability. An investigation into balance and shoe thickness from Canada showed that men aged between 60 and 82 kept better balance when wearing thin-soled shoes than when wearing thick-soled ones. The evidence came to light only when the men were asked to walk along a beam measuring 7.8 cm wide resting on pads on the floor. The critical area of the shoe was the "midsole," the foam-wedged section between the uppers and thin outersole. Most sports shoes have a midsole that yields too much to give stability. Softness may be comfortable, but it is not sufficiently supportive. The only sports shoe recommended in this report were those found to have a midsole density of "A 50," the hardest available. Manufacturers rarely state midsole specifications however. The researchers found similar results with women, and they recommend thin-soled, well-supporting shoes for walking, and never soft-soled slippers or bare feet for anyone not too steady on their feet.

- At any time in the day, stretch your toes from time to time and wiggle them about.

- The nail of the big toe may become thickened with age, making cutting difficult. Cut nails after bathing as water softens them. Bad cases may mean nail removal or filing the nail to manageable thickness. Get professional advice.

DIGESTION

Upset stomach, heartburn, dyspepsia, flatulence, gastritis, nausea and excess acid are all words used to describe symptoms of indigestion. Sufferers average four attacks a month according to one survey, and women are more vulnerable than men.

The most common remedies are over-the-counter neutralizing antacids, *prolonged use* of which can seriously harm heart, kidneys and bones. Antacids contain sodium (i.e., high salt content, which could be a hazard for anyone with high blood pressure), or calcium, magnesium, aluminum or simethicone, which is a gastric "defoaming" agent that breaks up gas bubbles.

Aluminum can cause constipation; magnesium in large amounts can cause diarrhea and tiredness; sodium bicarbonate can produce bloating and belching. Find the antacid that suits you best and read the label to see what you're getting.

Along with the harmful side effects listed above, there is the question mark hovering over aluminum in connection with Alzheimer's disease (see page 103). Anyone taking other medicines, or suffering from kidney problems, chronic bowel problems, or indeed any other chronic ailment, should consult a doctor before taking antacids.

For most people, occasional use is fine. Antacids should give relief within minutes. If symptoms persist, see your doctor.

The drug cimetidine, marketed as Tagamet, is now widely available, and reduces stomach acid very effectively, providing relief from symptoms for up to six hours. Again, discuss with your doctor if you need to use it regularly.

Ways to prevent indigestion:

- Don't eat big meals. Eat small ones more frequently and you'll give your stomach less work to do.

- Eat more slowly—again it's easier on the stomach.

- Don't lie down right after eating, especially after consuming fatty foods. Fat slows down stomach emptying and can encourage regurgitation or heartburn, with stomach acid coming up into the esophagus. If you're prone to heartburn, wait three hours before lying down, and then prop up with extra pillows when you do.

DUODENAL ULCERS

Duodenal ulcers are often inappropriately treated. Instead of the costly modern ulcer drugs, which heal ulcers but cannot stop them from recurring, inexpensive antibiotics could be used to better effect, says Dr. Kenneth McColl of the Western Infirmary in Glasgow. A three-week course of antibiotics can eliminate the H. pylori bacteria in the stomach that are the cause of at least 60 percent of ulcers.

- Don't eat a large meal or fatty foods late at night. When you go to sleep, the digestive system slows down, making a late, large meal seem to "stay in the stomach" long into the night.

- Comfortable clothes help digestion. Tight clothes constrict the stomach, causing discomfort and possibly heartburn.

- Caffeine, citrus fruits and tomatoes all make the stomach produce more acid, so watch for symptoms and cut down as necessary. Orange juice may be more of a problem than are fresh oranges.

- Try to prop up the top half of your bed if you get that burning feeling at night.

PROSTATE PROBLEMS

A very common problem for older men is difficulty in urinating. In most cases, this is due to an enlargement of the prostate gland, an organ that sits under the bladder and around the urethra, the channel through which urine passes. Enlargement obviously stops the flow. Despite greater awareness of the condition, and successful new treatments, many men remain remarkably shy about seeking professional help over this. Prevention is not possible, but all the general self-help measures may improve things. This includes reducing alcohol, tea and coffee, stopping smoking and increasing exercise. On the alternative medicine front, claims have been made about the extract of saw palmetto, a North American palm said to reduce symptoms, along with zinc, magnesium and various vitamins. Health food shops will stock a "cocktail" of such nutrients, but recognizing the symptoms and getting professional help early makes more sense. An enlarged prostate may be a sign of prostate cancer.

The typical symptoms:

- Difficulty or delay in starting to urinate
- Coming to a stop halfway through
- A weak stream that takes longer than it used to
- A follow-up trickle after finishing
- A feeling of not quite having emptied the bladder
- Going more often, including getting up at night

Even if any of these symptoms happen only occasionally, a checkup is worthwhile. Blood tests used to screen for prostate cancer can also help diagnose an enlarged prostate.

STRESS URINARY INCONTINENCE

This one is usually a "women's problem," often beginning in midlife and worsening with age. Symptoms are involuntary leaking of urine and the need to urinate frequently. Coughing or laughing can trigger involuntary leaking. The cause may go back to strain or injury in childbirth or muscle weakening and tissue-shrinking after menopause. Pelvic floor muscle exercises recommended before and after childbirth, also known as Kegel exercises, can help prevent the problem.

If the condition develops to the point where it gets out of control, a pro-lapse of the uterus or bladder may be the result, with surgery needed to repair it. But there should be no need to let things get that far. Estrogen replacement can help prevent bladder weakness by retaining tissue. There's also a new technique involving a collagen implant at the mouth of the bladder to help control leakage. But the exercises could stop the need for such measures, and may be as good as any drug therapy. When a group of 157 women aged from 55 to 90 were assigned either the exercises or a drug that contracts blood vessels in the bladder, the exercisers reported as much improvement in bladder control as did those taking the drug. But why wait until the condition develops? Pelvic floor exercises are good for everyone.

Exercises and safeguards:

- The basic pelvic floor exercise goes like this: Imagine you want to pass urine and tighten up the muscles as if to prevent it. You should feel the vagina pulling up at the same time.

- Hold this position for a few seconds, and then release.

- Repeat the exercise any time and anywhere. The women in the trial above were advised to repeat 80 times a day.

- When passing urine, try to stop the flow for a few seconds. Repeat once or twice. It may be difficult to do at first but perfor-mance quickly improves.

- Retrain your bladder by "holding on" rather than rushing to a toilet at the slightest urge. A longer hold each day helps strengthen the muscles.

- Bladder infections can occur after menopause when body tissue becomes thinner and less elastic. Urinate before and after sex, drink plenty of fluids, and don't let the bladder remain full for long periods even if you are "retraining."

ACHES AND ARTHRITIS

There are several forms of arthritis, and the one that's particularly com-mon in aging is osteoarthritis. You get pain and stiffness in joints, espe-cially those that take body weight—knees, hips, spine—but the fingers, wrists and neck are also commonly affected. The cause is mainly wear and tear, though being overweight, a previous injury or genetic predisposition are also factors. Around 9 percent of men and 14 percent of women will develop osteoarthritis of the knee because they are overweight. With age, the body simply does not produce enough of the thin film of lubrication, called synovial

> *Asked where she got her energy from at the age of 75, Eleanor Roosevelt, widow of the great president, said, "Part of it is in not getting too self-absorbed. Sure, there are aches and pains, but if you pay attention to them, you become an invalid."*

fluid, that cushions joints where they are in contact with each other. The resulting friction causes the pain and stiffness. Aspirin and other drugs can reduce pain and inflammation. Cures don't exist, despite many claims from the alternative medicine front, though oily fish or fish oil (see page 57) may help alleviate symptoms. An antibiotic, doxycycline, is being tested to see if it will halt the progress of the condition. Surgery to replace a hip or knee with an artificial joint may be a possible treatment once your joint is worn out.

If it's not the joints, it's the muscles, a common source of body pain that can come with age. Sitting for too long in one position, tension, intense concentration or sleeping in an awkward position are all likely causes.

Preventing aches and pains:

- Exercise won't guarantee an osteoarthritis-free future, but it helps. Try yoga, stretching exercises or swimming.
- Keep your weight down to decrease wear and tear on knee joints.
- Jogging and jumping put strain on joints—not the best exercise to prevent arthritis.
- Don't sit for too long in one position, when reading or watching television for instance. Standing, stretching and moving around reduce the chance of stiffness.
- Wear scarves, hats and other protective clothing to avoid the cold and drafts that can cause muscle stiffness and subsequent immobility.
- Keep warm in winter. Have a sauna or Turkish bath to bring heat to the bones and aid muscle relaxation.

CHAPTER FOUR

The Challenge of Looking Good

A QUESTION OF KEEPING UP APPEARANCES

Most of us would admit that we want to look good for our age, which is not at all the same as wanting to look our age. The real ambition, rather harder to acknowledge, is to look young for our age. We know how we looked at 40 or 50 or 60, and we would like to stop the clock there or there or there, anywhere younger than where we are now.

Being very elderly may not be so difficult once you've arrived. It's the getting there that can be so off-putting. We have to run the gauntlet of middle age, a time in which we have no aesthetic standard by which to judge ourselves, beyond the standard of youth. We are, by that standard, a failure. (Even the expression "middle age" has become uncomfortable. Instead we have "baby boomers.") The very old are at least allowed to be characterful, their past etched in their faces, so we fancifully like to think. Those in between who do not conform to youthful ideals are censured for failing to achieve an appropriate target.

Despite protests against being brainwashed by sexist ideas and commercial interests, women continue to starve themselves in order to look what they perceive to be smarter and younger. They are aware of, and want to avoid, the condemnation in that phrase "hasn't she put on weight," and the censoriousness in "hasn't she let herself go."

From their earliest days, women are aware of being scrutinized. Little girls in party dresses and cute hairdos, Hollywood close-ups showing every pore, advertisements revealing smooth, taut, unblemished flesh. The tyranny is unending. We are programmed to seek perfection and deny the reality of our aging, sagging, wrinkling bodies.

When do we stop caring and competing for youthful looks, and accept that we are "old"? It's quite possible that we never do. Looking good is so tied up with looking younger that we may never quite be able to separate the two, and the 90-year-old woman who goes to the hairdresser, or her male counterpart who takes care to arrange his hair to cover his bald patch, may be seeking to play their idea of sprightly 80 year olds, and to hell with the tasteful facial character lines. Everything is relative.

This should be cheering news. Being any age, once we arrive at it, is not so bad after all. We can settle for this amount of wrinkles, that amount of sagging. As a species we are eminently adaptable, we can get used to things, find ways of accommodating reality. It's only the future that we hate, the changes-to-be that we dread, the stuff we have not yet experienced that we fear.

We have ways of fighting these things of course. With money and nerve, we can go for the nips and tucks and suctions of cosmetic surgery. We can select esoteric creams and lotions, beauty therapies, exercises for face and body that promise, not always truthfully, to shape and smooth and sculpt and turn back the clock.

These are not the only choices. We can learn to invest less in looks, make a compromise, skim over these features, emphasize those, develop a dispassionate response to aging contours of face and body, be proud of our wrinkles. We can deny the whole process, look in the mirror and gloss over what we see, pretending nothing has happened to make our faces match our years. Even our best friends won't tell us.

What most of us do is a bit of everything. We make efforts to look young, or good. We think of face creams and makeup as enhancing accessories, the way we think of a new outfit or hairdo. We also, most of us, acknowledge our aging images in the mirror, but at times "edit out" what we don't want to see.

And for what do we do these things? The question can be answered in several ways. Do we do it for love, approval, attention? If these are the reasons, then our post-Freudian understanding would suggest that they signify fear of change and lack of confidence in growing older. Is another motive to compensate for being ignored, overlooked and lacking credibility? If so, we can add ageism and sexism as highly influential reasons. Or is a major reason for keeping up appearances that we feel positive and can celebrate a zest for life? Not all responses have to be negative (people suffering from depression don't usually care about their appearance).

We don't have to be victims of ageism or sexism or exploitative commercialism, which play on our fear of change, when we invest in face or body enhancement. We can choose how far we want to go, whether it's trying anti-aging creams or cosmetic surgery or allowing nature to take its course unaided.

Since the opportunities exist, and few of us resist them entirely, the following pages provide information and ideas on what can be done to preserve what we've got. Some of them work better in mind than in body—the feel-good factor gets going the minute we start doing something positive. But first and foremost comes basic body health, which is, we are now finding, inseparable from shape and size.

WHAT YOUR SHAPE TELLS YOU

The subject of losing weight and keeping slim is loaded with both sexual politics and science. We now know that it is not so much how fat you are as where the fat is, a truism that applies to health as well as aesthetics. Scientists have discovered a great deal in the last few years about the way body shape can predict certain diseases. Psychologists are finding that dissatisfaction about body image works very differently in men and women. And feminists are deploring the emphasis on unnatural slimness in fashion and advertising, and the recurring image of nymphs and waifs and anorexic lookalikes promoted as an ideal for the female shape.

Being a little overweight in midlife and old age may actually be good for you according to some studies, but the overall evidence is that as Western populations put on weight, they increase their risk of falling victim to elevated blood pressure, diabetes, high cholesterol levels, gall-bladder disease and cancers. A long-term investigation of the incidence of fatal heart disease in relation to obesity in 116,000 women concluded that being even mildly to moderately overweight increased the risk of heart disease in middle-aged women.

The long-term Heart Disease Epidemiology Study in Framingham, Massachusetts, found obesity to be a clear marker for heart disease in women and men, but pinpointed central obesity, the apple shape, as being especially significant, particularly in men. This study also found increased death rates in the thinnest members of the population, especially older men.

Another major piece of research came to a different conclusion, claiming that thinness is best, especially in middle-aged men (this dovetails with the low-calorie/life extension theory explained earlier). Not if they smoke, though. While cigarette smokers are generally leaner than nonsmokers, they don't get the built-in benefit of a longer life span.

THE APPLE SHAPE

The picture, then, is not clear, but the new findings on body shape provide some useful clues. It looks as if a thickened waistline is not good news for men or women in middle age. Five years of investigation by Dr. Aaron Folsom and his team at the University of Minnesota's School of Public Health have led to the conclusion that the bigger the waist compared with the hips, the greater the danger of ill health in later life. Women aged 55 to 69 with a dangerously small waist-hip ratio have a 60 percent increased risk of dying prematurely. From a health point of view, the ideal shape for women is a waist less than 80 percent of hips—for example, 40-inch hips and 32-inch waist. For men, the ideal ratio is 95 percent.

How do people acquire an apple shape or the risky 20 percent above average weight for their height? A sedentary life and too much eating and drinking are not the only reasons. Heredity has a lot to do with it.

When 12 pairs of identical male twins, observed in a study at Quebec's Laval University, ate an extra 1000 calories for six days a week for 100 days, they appeared to use those extra calories in very different ways. Some pairs of twins gained 9 pounds each in weight, while other pairs gained up to 29 pounds. Each pair gained the same amount, and in the same places. Those who gained less were assumed to use many of the extra calories in building muscle tissue. The ones who gained more did what other weight-gainers do: their fat cells expanded and multiplied to store the fat from the extra calories that were surplus to their energy needs. This discouraging finding, from the *New England Journal of Medicine*, suggests that the genetic factor is as least as strong as diet or lifestyle. Another piece of research from Sweden showed that identical twins raised apart have similar body weights.

BODY FACTS

• Lean body mass is greater in men than in women of all ages, including infancy, but in both sexes it declines with age.

• Body fat distribution changes in women and men with age, with less subcutaneous fat under the skin, and more internal fat, much of it in the abdominal area.

• Women in their 60s have narrower shoulders, broader hips and wider chests than women in their 20s.

• Changes in body composition, with loss of fluid, fat and calcium, plus muscle atrophy, lead to weight loss in the very old. In some women, this weight loss begins at around 50.

• The taller you are, up to 6 feet 2 inches, the greater your chances of long life—due, it is thought, to nutritional development in the womb and in infancy.

Central obesity, as the apple shape is called, may well be inherited, and indicates that the owners of this phenomenon, male and female, lay down a different kind of fat to that found in other parts of the body. This body fat is more common after menopause, when women begin to catch up with men in heart disease risk, and it appears to have a harmful effect on hormones, insulin, cholesterol and HDL and LDL levels in the blood.

The solution is not liposuction or other cosmetic surgery to remove the offending fat, but controlled, gradual dieting, healthy foods and plenty of exercise. Many scientists today claim that body fat in other areas is harmless except in cases of extreme obesity, which means that if you are a wide-hipped pear or a curvy hourglass, you can safely carry several excess pounds. But not too many. Obesity is still reckoned to be 20 percent or more of weight above the ideal.

HOW WE FEEL ABOUT HOW WE LOOK

Few researchers take an interest in middle-aged views on body image, but Paul Rozin and April Fallon, of the University of Pennsylvania, compared two generations—fathers and sons plus mothers and daughters—on how they felt about their appearance. The mothers and daughters were more concerned about weight and diet than the fathers and sons, which was to be expected. Even so, many of the fathers perceived themselves as being as far from an ideal weight as the women of both generations.

An investigation of 87 American college women and 118 college men confirmed earlier studies that women overestimate male preferences for thin female figures. When shown a range of silhouettes, 69 percent of the women regarded the three thinnest as most attractive to men, but only 25 percent of the men selected these, thus confirming that women opt for the fashion image, while men go for the sensual and curvy.

More unexpected was the finding that the women also chose a very slim silhouette as the kind they thought other women would find attractive, but when asked to select a silhouette that pleased themselves, they chose something a bit more realistic. In this case their "desirable" silhouette was more curvy though still thinner than their own body weight. Only 6 percent of the women described themselves as "very fat," yet 24 percent wished to be "a lot thinner."

When men were asked to judge the male shape that they thought other men would admire, they selected large physiques. Choosing an ideal for themselves, in general they chose silhouettes that were near to the way they were and did not share a single definition of an ideal figure. But they must have had some ideals in mind, since around one-third wanted to be thinner, and slightly more than that wanted to be "heavier."

Men can also get it wrong when it comes to choosing the shape they think will attract the opposite sex. Muscularity has emerged in research as a major concern to men, with underweight college men viewing themselves negatively. But women are not too concerned about muscularity in men, and in surveys have shown that they actually prefer men with thinner physiques.

THE WEIGHT DEBATE— GOOD AND BAD DIETING

"When a person gains weight and stays that weight a while, the body will defend that weight. It becomes the new 'set point.' " The words are those of Xavier Pi-Sunyer of the Obesity Research Center at St. Luke's–Roosevelt Hospital in New York, and they come as no great surprise. It seems that our bodies stubbornly resist our efforts to reduce their size, and they employ a number of different mechanisms to do so.

For a start, dieting slows the metabolic rate, making calories burn less speedily. And as the fat cells shrink, they are programmed by insulin to release their contents more slowly, too.

Another form of sabotage is an enzyme called LPL (for lipoprotein lipase), produced by fat cells to help store calories as fat. We can, through inherited genes, produce too much LPL and be especially efficient at storing calories. When LPL levels were measured in nine people who had lost weight, the levels had risen. They rose most in the people who had been fattest before dieting, and the researchers, reporting in the *New England Journal of Medicine*, concluded that the LPL enzyme was working overtime to get the body back to its former weight.

This LPL is thought to be partially controlled by estrogen in women and testosterone in men. Fat cells in women secrete LPL in hips, thighs and breasts. The waist and midriff area is the focus of LPL in men.

> *"In Sierra Leone where I worked for two years, there was a view that God gave you your body—fatness, thinness, a limp were all God-given. So there was less obsession about appearance or the need to change your body."*
>
> *—Aid worker on her experience in Africa.*

Maybe this accounts for the fact that men and women lose fat at different rates. Fat from cells in the abdominal area can be released quickly for energy when needed. Fat deposited in thighs and buttocks is used for long-term storage.

So far, so bad. It looks as if dieting is a waste of time. Not true, but it's all a question of how. The yo-yo dieting lifestyle—lose and gain, lose and gain, again and again—is positively unhealthy. Body weight fluctuation, often repeated or great, is linked with a higher risk of heart disease and death. This may be due to the effect of dieting on cholesterol levels, which rise during periods of loss and gain.

One piece of research on this comes from the long-term Framingham study now going for over 30 years. Weight fluctuation was found most in the younger part of the population studied, those aged between 30 and 44 years (though there is no reason to think that older people have a different pattern). The critical fluctuation is thought to be 11 pounds or more. Being a bit overweight consistently is safer than yo-yo dieting, say researchers, and they recommend the importance of maintaining weight loss. If you can keep weight off for two years, you're likely to keep it off for good.

THE BEST KIND OF DIET

Forget the crash diet or the very low calorie diet. They seriously decrease body strength so if you try to do the healthy thing and exercise at the same time, you won't have the muscle power for it. These diets also do nothing about changing long-term eating patterns and often re-

> *The safe way to lose weight and not regain it is to re-educate eating habits and to get regular exercise. You eat less fat, wean yourself off sugary foods, and you learn to live on fewer calories for good.*

inforce a taste for sweet foods since many are themselves sweet. Forget special combination diets, detoxification diets and one-food diets. If there is anything in the idea that particular foods or combinations are extra-effective for weight loss for certain people, they'd need individual testing and monitoring to find out. Forget spot dieting methods that claim to attack cellulite and work magic on a specific area. They're an illusion. You lose weight gradually in all areas, starting with the middle of the body and the abdomen. Hips and thighs may seem to reduce quickly, but that's more likely to be the toning effect of exercising.

The fat-sugar cutback has more to offer than reducing calories indiscriminately. There are, it seems from new research, calories and calories. Virtually all of those derived from fat go into immediate storage in the fat cells. Carbohydrates and protein convert into glucose for energy, with only that in excess of body needs being stored. The most healthy and effective gradual diet is one that cuts fat intake to 20 percent, allowing energy requirements to be met by carbohydrates and protein. Overweight people may be getting 35 percent of their calories from fat.

Exercise is the other aid to weight loss. It not only helps by burning off calories, it boosts the rate of calorie burn-off for several hours afterward. There's no need to go to excess though. Moderate aerobic exercise will work.

There is no need for excessive food deprivation either. A gradual weight loss will last longer than the short, sharp treatment, and be safer from a health point of view.

SEVEN WAYS TO CHANGE YOUR EATING HABITS

1. If you haven't done so already, give up adding sugar to your tea and coffee. It's easier than you may think, and is the beginning of acquiring a taste for less sweet foods.

2. Before cutting into the cake, just remember this: 4 ounces of chocolate cake provides 555 calories and 39.3 g sugars. The same amount of banana provides 79 calories and 16.2 g sugar, and 100 g of apple contains only 46 calories and 11.8 g sugars. So when you yearn for something sweet, eat a piece of fresh fruit first. Enjoy the natural sweetness and don't ask for anything more.

3. Dried fruit can satisfy a sweet tooth from time to time. Here's what you get: 4 dried dates = 148 calories and 28.8 g sugars; a small handful of raisins or sultanas (15 g) = 37 calories and 9.7 g sugars. Compare this with a 100 g milk chocolate bar = 529 calories and 56.5 g sugars.

4. You know the danger times for snacks—mid-morning, mid-afternoon, late evening. Get into the habit of having handy some low-fat yogurt, cucumber, grated carrot in a little low-fat dressing or orange juice, or a rice cake, and choose from these instead of chips, nuts or sweet snacks at the tempting moments.

5. A gram of fat has 9 calories; a gram of carbohydrate or protein has only 4. So you get more on your plate when it is piled with carbohydrates or protein—a large baked potato has, for instance, the same number of calories as 42 g (1.5 oz) of potato chips, both being about 225 calories.

CAN CENTRAL HEATING MAKE YOU FAT?

Scientists in Cambridge, England, are researching the possibility that getting out into the cold increases the metabolic rate to keep the body warm and is therefore a way of spending calories. Staying indoors on a cold day without central heating could do the same. Critics of the theory say that it would have to be very cold indeed to affect metabolic rate. But true or false, the exercise in itself can only do good. One piece of consolation for female dieters: women are able to withstand the cold more effectively than men because even when slim they have a thicker layer of subcutaneous fat.

6. Eating on social occasions means inevitable lapses. Enjoy but be a little more frugal for the next day or two.

7. Buy low-fat foods, low-fat or nonfat milk and low-sugar drinks—preferably fresh fruit juices. Switch to nonsweetened breakfast cereal and think how many calories you save when combining it with skimmed milk. Check the calorie content of foods described as "lite." They may be only a very little lighter than ordinary foods, and may contain more sugar although less fat.

DIETING DELUSIONS

- We eat less butter and more nonfat milk, and the extra fat goes into ice cream. Sales in ice cream are booming.

- We tend to underestimate the amount of calories we take in, glossing over the odd 50 here and there and arriving at a figure that can be 50 percent less than the truth.

- We tend to allow ourselves "just a little more" when we have exercised or detect a small fall in weight. Immediate dramatic weight loss tends to be from fluid, which is equally speedily replaced.

- Eating on the run may seem like low food intake, but snacks are often high in fats and sugar, containing more calories than a proper meal.

- While we virtuously avoid the sweets and chocolates when perusing the shopping aisles, come the check-out line, with those tempting last-minute displays, and we're all too often lost.

SIX WAYS TO RECOGNIZE
WHEN YOUR DIETING IS GETTING OUT OF HAND

1. You eat separately from the family.

2. You eat little when with other people and then rush to the refrigerator for something the minute you're alone.

3. You go in for binges—like a whole pack of cookies or several chocolate bars at one sitting.

4. You turn down invitations because you fear abandoning your diet.

5. You find yourself thinking about food a lot of the time.

6. You push yourself harder and harder when exercising in order to work off calories.

If you feel guilty or anxious or depressed when you lapse, the reason may be chemical, not psychological. A psychiatrist at Manchester Royal Infirmary in England has found that weight-reducing diets can disrupt the functioning of the neurotransmitter serotonin. The disruption can make sticking to a diet impossible because of mood swings, irritability, depression, anxiety or uncontrollable hunger—all due to a reduced output of serotonin in the brain. Women may be more affected than men, which could account for more eating disorders in women. This finding is leading to new treatments. Instead of the traditional antidepressants to treat eating disorders, a drug called fluoxetine, which enhances serotonin function, is on trial in the United States, Canada and the United Kingdom, and has showed good results with sufferers of bulimia, though it will probably work best when combined with counseling.

THE FUTURE IN MAGIC PILLS

Metabolism-altering drugs are not an illusion. Pharmaceutical companies are spending millions on exploring what could be the Holy Grail of dieting.

One type of drug known as an amylin blocker could stop the onset of diabetes by controlling blood glucose levels, and it may also one day act as a slimming pill. Another drug, THT, or tetra-hydrolipstatin, may one day help seriously overweight people by preventing absorption of fat in the diet. However, THL could deprive the body of important health-giving fats and may have potential risks. It could go the way of appetite suppressants, many of which have been found unacceptable because they cause dependency, increase blood pressure or have other undesirable side effects. The magic pill is still a long way off.

THE SKIN TRADE—PROMISES, PROMISES

"Major advances" or "breakthrough" developments are the kinds of phrases that come out from skin-care industry ads, and we have heard them all before. We are used to being served up vaguely scientific explanations and promises to preserve youth and protect skin from the ravages of time.

Nowadays, men as well as women are being wooed by sophisticated anti-aging products that have the blessing of highly respectable dermatologists and, in some cases, the Food and Drug Administration (FDA) approval. Whatever the promises, they have a lot to overcome.

To take the aging process alone—as we age, our skin becomes dryer, thinner and less elastic. This is due to the sebaceous, grease-producing glands becoming less efficient and collagen and elastin losing their ability to support the skin cells and maintain flexibility and elasticity. From about the age of 60, skin cell replacement slows downs and the outer layer of cells are retained longer so the skin looks duller. The free radicals that age the rest of our bodies do their worst here, too. On top of this, our aging complexions have to deal with cigarette smoke, air pollution and a lifetime's exposure to sunlight, which may do the worst damage of all.

ANTI-AGING CREAMS—DO THEY WORK?

Anti-aging creams can only do so much, and it may not in fact be all that much despite the hyperbole. A smoother skin, fainter lines, but nothing spectacular, seems to be the verdict of many who have tried them. Some product photographs show convincing and dramatic changes around the eyes, where puffiness and deep wrinkles are noticeably reduced. Sagging and wrinkled jawlines don't do so well, presumably because they have more to contend with on the gravity front. The skin of a 40 year old does better and gets faster results than does older skin.

The big change with new anti-aging skin products is the acknowledgment that they can penetrate the skin. This means they are recognized as a drug. As a result, some are applying for FDA approval.

All products designed to improve the skin must be used continuously, which means big business for those who make and market them. Most consumers today are sophisticated and cynical enough to take any miracle claims of effectiveness with a pinch of salt. And yet we do hope for miracles, just very tiny ones—otherwise why would we bother to buy the stuff and put it on with fairly faithful regularity?

One thing we can do without is the approach found all too often in promotional material and designed to make the hesitant or unwilling consumer feel guilty, fearful and even irresponsible. "You owe it to yourself to take advantage of modern products," is how the psychology goes. Here's a prime example: "The wrinkle is a serious disease. Do you know anybody who gets up every morning and worries about illness? But everybody worries regularly about wrinkles." This quote is printed in publicity material for the anti-aging skin treatment Tretinoin. It is attributed to Professor Albert Kligman who introduced the drug, originally used for acne.

That said, the major developments promising minor "miracles" are reaching a wide public. Meanwhile, cosmetic companies race for new and improved versions, proof, if ever we needed it, that the best we've got still leaves much to be desired. Here are three major recently developed types of anti-aging skin products:

AHA, OR ALPHA HYDROXY ACIDS

These are promoted as new by beauty-product companies, but have actually been known to dermatologists as a treatment for acne and warts long before they became fashionable for anti-aging. They derive from sugar cane, fruits and milk, and they work by speeding up the removal of a natural substance that holds dead cells on the skin. The acceleration in cell turnover reveals a fresher, smoother layer of skin, with a texture that appears fine and more light-reflecting—in other words younger. There are claims that AHAs increase moisture-holding ability and stimulate collagen production as well as reducing fine lines.

There are different strengths of AHAs. Over-the-counter products—often their names or descriptions include the word fruit on them—are less concentrated than those used in beauty salons, and they stay in the superficial layers of the skin, so the peeling effect is not too deep and any stinging reaction which can occur with these products is usually only temporary. Deep peels done in a doctor's office can cause stinging, swelling, even weeping sores which can take weeks or months to clear. They also produce better results in appearance once the agony is over.

Retin-A

The big star before AHAs came along, Retin-A is still the one that best restores sun-damaged skin. The substance is a derivative of vitamin A, and is sometimes used by dermatologists to treat acne. It can reduce the so-called "liver spots" (groups of darker pigment cells caused by sun exposure and aging), speed cell turnover and may boost collagen production. Redness, skin flaking and oversensitivity to sunlight are common side effects of the full-strength treatment, which can be obtained only through a doctor's prescription. Milder versions are available but tend to be less effective, though new powerful variations being developed may produce less redness.

Antioxidant Nutrient Creams and Gels

These are more gentle treatments that claim to combat free radicals and rejuvenate tired skin. Consisting mostly of vitamins, they contradict the traditional view that vitamins in face creams would do more for you if you ate them. Now we are offered vitamins C and E and gamma linolenic acid, the substance contained in evening primrose oil, as ways to restore sun-damaged skin, replace collagen, fight free radicals and produce a fine, firmer appearance of the skin. Cellex-C (the "C" as in vitamin C) is a new product being developed by Dr. Lorraine Meisner of the University of Wisconsin, Madison. Dr. Meisner admits that her product works best on shallow wrinkles, but is convinced it does work. At the moment, it is being tested for FDA approval.

Face Savers to Swallow

Eating antioxidants in the form of fresh fruit and vegetables forms the best basis of beauty-from-within. No one, however, would claim that doing so will remove wrinkles in three months, as sellers of beauty pills claim about their products.

These pills are usually a cocktail of vitamins and/or minerals to be taken daily as a food supplement. One product contains a witch's brew consisting of "extract of natural marine organisms with vitamin and mineral co-factors" that includes shrimp cells, underwater plants

Even without full sunshine, beware of damage from sun exposure. When it's cloudy but still bright, those destructive rays can get at you. Always use a sunblock of at least SPF (skin protection factor) 15.

and fish cartilage. The publicity material states that after three months of daily use, thickness and elasticity improved in 15 women with a mean age of 50 when they were compared with another group of 15 women on a placebo pill. Wrinkles lessened in the treated group and brittle hair and nails also improved. Despite claims from some dermatologists of similarly impressive results, and newspaper claims that these findings would be published in the *British Journal of Dermatology*, as of yet no paper has been accepted.

DON'T LET THE SUN SHINE IN

It's called photoaging, not just aging—the process initiated by sunlight that makes the skin less elastic. Collagen and elastin, the proteins that give skin elasticity, are damaged. Enzymes that break down these proteins increase. Upper-layer skin cells, keratinocytes, which are shed and renewed more slowly with age, are also damaged by photoaging. Other skin cells, melanocytes, are killed by it.

Even without full sunshine, beware of damage from sun exposure. When it's cloudy but still bright, those destructive rays can get at you. Always use a sunblock of at least SPF (skin protection factor) 15, or choose a moisturizer or foundation with sunscreens.

Ordinary clothing may not offer enough protection. If you spend long periods in the sun and have fine, fair skin that burns easily, you could get burned through ordinary clothes, even when they are of tightly woven fabric like cotton jersey. Anyone needing extra protection—and that includes anyone who's had any form of abnormal mole or skin cancer—should look into densely woven protective clothing, available at some sporting goods stores and by mail order.

MORE FACTS ON SKIN

- Women get the short straw yet again, with skin aging extra quickly at menopause. But even before that they have more wrinkles than men. Professor Shabtay Dikstein in Jerusalem found ways to measure skin suppleness and moisture, and found that women aged 20 to 40 had 40 percent more wrinkles than men, while females age 60 and over had 75 percent more wrinkles than men.

- Hormone replacement therapy (HRT) is known to thicken skin and improve appearance—though for many years the medical profession said the effect was merely in the eye of the user. Evidence from one study supports the idea that HRT maintains or enhances collagen, giving skin elasticity and firmness. It seems that two kinds of collagen exist in human skin, and proportions change rapidly after menopause. HRT can help put the balance right.

- Exercise can help the skin by treating it to extra oxygen. Through regular physical activity, oxygen boosts circulation, making the body work more efficiently at draining lymph nodes and flushing away toxins.

- The best moisturizer ever is petroleum jelly, the most popular brand being Vaseline™, long recommended by dermatologists. Not too nice to use, and too heavy for under the eyes, but a great help when the skin feels extra dry as it keeps natural moisture in. It may even be absorbed into the skin and protect against ultraviolet light, according to recent research from university medical schools in San Francisco and Pennsylvania.

- Passive smoking is damaging to the skin. Researchers at Estee Lauder Cosmetics found that smokers and those in close contact lost skin moisture more rapidly than did nonsmokers. To compensate, new products are being developed that contain antioxidants which neutralize free radicals specific to cigarette smoke.

- The skin around the eyes is the thinnest anywhere on the body. Some moisturizers can be too much for it, causing a stinging or burning sensation. Eye gels are light, soothing and act as a gentle moisturizer.

- The dryness and skin thinning that come with aging can have some literally irritating effects such as an increased sensitivity to detergents, wool, and even to some drugs. A skin rash reaction to drugs can take as long as a month to appear.

THE NATURAL FACELIFT

Do facial exercises help? "Smile a lot—that will exercise your muscles," said one doctor cynically. A yoga headstand will stimulate circulation, said an alternative practitioner. Don't massage facial skin after the age of 40, said a beautician. All good advice, and at least two of the tips should be easy to follow.

Claims for the benefits of facial exercises come mainly from the enthusiasts who devise them, follow them faithfully, look marvelous and publish books sharing their routines with the general public. If you care sufficiently and dedicate yourself to such routines, go buy one of the books and you too may see good results.

HAIR TODAY AND TOMORROW?

Our hair's quality is another sensitive area. Should we dye out the gray and try to restore lost hair, or should we accept the changes gracefully? The debate continues. Meanwhile here's some of the latest thinking:

- **A sure cure for thinning hair and baldness** is as elusive as a definitive skin rejuvenator. The hair restorer Rogaine®, based on the drug minoxidil, is at the time of writing the only product licensed to restore hair, and for some it works very well if applied to the scalp on a daily basis, though the longer the baldness has existed the less likely you are to see results. Hair-grafting replacement techniques can be painful and not always convincing, though laser methods being developed promise to bypass current problems such as uneven tufts, brown hairs and complications due to grafts and incisions. On the far horizon could be a genetic cure, as scientists are searching for what they believe is a gene for baldness.

- **Hair loss in women** is not unusual at menopause and later. The loss is usually gradual, either starting above the temples, or a thinning all over as hair follicles shrink. Body-building conditioners, gels and styling lotions puff out and thicken individual strands but can make them too stiff and heavy if large amounts are used. A good cut will help disguise thin patches, with minimum layering or a bob. Minoxidil or hair grafts work for women as well as men. Sometimes salon treatments, with hair tugged by stylists, add to the problem of hair loss. Washing hair at home using mild shampoo and keeping styling lotions to a minimum for six months can help.

- **Facial hair on women** tends to increase after menopause, and the best permanent way to remove it is still electrolysis, a process which takes time as each regrowth has to be treated until the hair is very fine. Tweezing out hairs and depilatory creams can produce a bristly regrowth.

- **Hair dyes, how safe?** The jury is still out on the link between hair colorings and cancer. Recently a link has been made between men using hair dyes and bone-marrow cancer. There may be a connection between prolonged use of a certain color hair dye and Hodgkins' lymphoma and multiple myeloma. The advice to men is the same as to women: use henna or colorants that coat the hair and wash out. It's the permanent dyes, which penetrate the hair and scalp, that could be dangerous.

BODY SCULPTURE— EVERYTHING THAT MONEY CAN BUY

You don't have to be rich and famous to have cosmetic surgery, so the practitioners and their publicists tell us. Famous maybe not, but we're still talking serious money. You also need a strong nerve, and that's not only for the hefty bills. An anesthetic, possibly pain, a period of weeks or months when the skin is swollen or bruised, a risk of mistakes or complications and no guarantee that you'll get precisely what you hope for all mean that you have to be pretty optimistic and highly motivated to hand over your body and your bank account.

What you get is not instant youth. This is definitely feel-good territory once the bruises and scars have healed. There is no great dramatic change in looks, which is just as well when one thinks about it. But subtle smoothers and shapers, fat removers and redistributors can work for almost any part of the body. Some procedures can be done as an outpatient at a clinic using a local anesthetic; others may require a hospital stay and a general anesthetic.

Check out the surgeon's background and references before you go ahead with any treatment. Also ask for a computer image to demonstrate the effect of proposed improvements, and discuss your skin type. The darker the skin color, the greater chance of noticeable scarring after a face-lift. Black skin can suffer keloids—thickened scar tissue—and pigment changes. Chemical peeling and dermabrasion again work best on the lightest-toned skins, with brunettes and darker skinned people possibly suffering skin discoloration or scarring.

SHOULD YOU, SHOULDN'T YOU?

No "should" about it, even if you have money, time and courage. Don't ever fall for the owe-it-to yourself school of hidden persuasion. "Everybody wants to be beautiful. People want to be seen," said one eminent surgeon, condemning in two short sentences the poor who can't afford his treatment, the "unreasonable" who refuse it and the elderly with their untreated, if not untreatable wrinkles who, according to his logic, are unfit to be seen.

One of the blessings of growing older is that we have the opportunity to liberate ourselves from the constraints of trying to be beautiful. We can learn to appreciate ourselves and others without reference to looks.

SURGERY TO HOLD BACK THE CLOCK

LIPOSUCTION

Removing fat by instruments that draw off fat cells is painless and fast. There's usually no need for a general anesthetic or overnight stay. The fat cells, once removed, don't come back, and abdomen, hips, thighs, upper arms, chins, even knees can have bulging fat suctioned away. Sounds simple—but it isn't, and it needs to be done by a fully qualified cosmetic surgeon. Sometimes the fat extraction is uneven, leaving a lumpy effect that is difficult to correct. Swelling and bruising can continue just as long as it occurs with traditional cosmetic surgery. There are other risks as well, including infection.

Liposuction may not be enough for aging skin and flesh. If a lot of fat is removed in people over 55, there is a high risk that the skin may sag and wrinkle. Almost certainly a tuck will be needed, too. Professor Pierre Fournier, who has developed a version called liposculpture, which he claims uses more sensitive contouring instruments, says it is effective on the face up to about the age of 55, but after that may need a little help from the surgeon's knife. Fat transfer, taking the unwanted cells and injecting them into, for instance, sagging cheeks, jawline, forehead or upper arms, fills out the areas hollowed by time and nature. Again, the treatment works better for younger than older skin. The effect can last a year or so.

THE FULL FACE-LIFT

This is no longer a "simple" case of lifting the top layer of skin. Now fat and muscle get shifted around, too, for a longer lasting and more natural look. Hollow cheeks can be filled out, excess skin on jowls can be removed, neck muscles tightened. Fat may be implanted into creases. A full face-lift can last ten years. Partial lifts are a waste of money, but there are other specific procedures as mentioned below.

CHEEK IMPLANTS

Loss of teeth, the effect of losing weight, and aging itself can make cheeks sag. At one time, silicone was used to restore contour, now it's more likely to be fat removed by liposuction from elsewhere in the body, or even a synthetic paste that can be molded onto the bone.

EYEBAG REMOVAL

Work on the eye area is called blepharoplasty. The surgeon makes a cut and takes away surplus skin just below lower lashes, or works similarly on upper lids. An eyebrow lift can also be performed to smooth out forehead wrinkles.

DOUBLE CHIN

The fat creating the double chin is removed by liposuction. Once it is gone it won't come back, but if skin lacks elasticity, a tuck may be needed, too.

ABDOMEN REDUCTION

The "tummy tuck" removes skin and fat, and muscles may be tightened at the same time. Liposuction to remove excess fats is often carried out as part of the process.

SKIN IMPROVERS

Chemical peeling with lactic acid (AHAs), Retin-A and/or dermabrasion techniques using fine abrasive brushes can remove scars, brown spots, fine wrinkles and rough skin surface. Collagen implants to fill out furrows and deep grooves look impressive to begin with but need a touch-up every few months. An asthma drug, aminophylline, can

LAST WORDS ON BEAUTY

Western culture programs us to hate our aging bodies, the flab, the thread veins, the loss of contour and smoothness. But we can learn to love our bodies for their vulnerability as we love the vulnerable undeveloped bodies of babies. The mending and patching of cosmetic surgery is ultimately a denial of the endurance and triumph of aging. To be proud of our imperfections must be the ultimate goal.

"melt" unwanted cellulite off thighs, though it does not work for everyone. A bacteria-derived toxin, botulin, freezes muscles and erases wrinkles for up to three months. A version of the fabric Gore-Tex™, threaded under the skin, fills wrinkles permanently. CACI (Computer Aided Cosmetology Instrument) is one of a number of techniques that use electrodes to contract facial muscles and soften wrinkles. These techniques require several initial treatments and four to six maintenance treatments a year. Acupressure and acupuncture make certain claims to create a more youthful appearance and may increase circulation and reduce "stress" lines.

COSMETIC DENTISTRY

Tooth-colored composite resin, porcelain veneers, tooth whiteners and gap-fillers are part of the repertoire of cosmetic dentistry. Resins can last up to eight years; veneers 15 or even 20. However, some dentists have a reputation of overselling their services.

CHAPTER FIVE

The Brain Challenge

AGE-PROOFING YOUR MIND

Sir John Gielgud, the celebrated Shakespearean actor, grumbled about the celebrations for his 90th birthday. "They are simply embarrassing," he is reported to have said. "All I want to do is to continue working." His motives may have been modesty or cussedness, but they make good sense. Working is clearly the secret of his successful longevity. Every time we fall for the idea that aging means getting dotty and forgetful, we should remember John Gielgud and realize that the human brain does not inevitably go into decline. The ability to remember lines, get to rehearsals, work with fellow actors, retain timing, judgment and emotional depth are all aspects of a working day in the life of an elderly actor.

HOW THE BRAIN AGES

Despite these achievements, brains do change with age. We lose brain cells, or *neurons*—around 50,000 of them a day over a lifetime. This may sound terrible but it works out at merely 3 percent of the total by the age of 80, since we start off with a good ten billion neurons. We also, over the years, lose some of the chemical messengers, or *neurotransmitters*, which carry information from one nerve cell to another.

But the brain works in mysterious ways. If one neuron fails, its neighbors can compensate. When Stanley Rapoport of the National Institutes of Health mapped neural networks in old and young people by measuring brain blood flow, he found that the networks took different paths in the different age groups, although performances were the same.

From about the age of 50, reaction time, memory, learning ability, problem-solving and decision-making may begin to decline. Blood supply to the brain can be reduced by 20 to 25 percent between the ages of 30 and 70. Reaction time, based on messages from brain to body, is thought to slow down by 30 to 40 percent. This means we will be slower to jam on the car's brakes when required or to hit a tennis ball at the crucial moment.

But again all is not what it seems. When different age groups are compared, there is a great overlap in ability. Ill health, genetic makeup and physical or mental inactivity contribute greatly to variation in performance in older people.

This is the way three eminent physicians—Nicholas Coni, William Davison and Stephen Webster—sum up the situation in their book, *Ageing—The Facts*:

> "There seems to be some decline in intellectual function which does not begin early, does not affect all aspects of the intelligence, and is not universal and inevitable in all the elderly. From the early 60s to the mid-70s, there is normally a decline in some but not all abilities in some but not all people. After the age of 80, however, a decline is the rule."

WHICH PEOPLE STAY MENTALLY YOUNGER LONGER?

We get some clues from rats. When deprived of stimulation, the brains of rats shrink, claims Marion Diamond of the University of California,

Berkeley. However, if the deprived rats are given a variety of toys, wheels and ladders and a month in the company of fellow rats, they gain extra blood supply in the brain and an increase in brain size.

The same may be true of aging humans. Those who regularly play bridge or do crossword puzzles score better in mental tests than those who rely on bingo to sharpen their wits. The use-it-or-lose-it dictum applies as much to mental as it does to physical power. In physically active older people, physical and mental reaction time has been found to match that of younger individuals.

So far, the inference is that you have to work at keeping mentally on top. But there are some ways in which getting older means getting better. Experience really does bring better judgment. If we slow down when making decisions, it is partly due to a desire for accuracy rather than speed. We know more and therefore need more time to think. We opt for the considered and careful and trust less in the hazardous hopeful. Similarly, the quick reaction of the young is often far from the ideal. An older driver who is slower to use the brakes is also less likely to need them in emergencies. Older people know when they feel tired and begin to lose attention. Their threshold may be lower than that of younger people, but they are more likely to give in gracefully than overstretch themselves.

Getting older can mean getting cleverer. When experienced typists of college age were compared with a similarly accurate group over 60, the young were expected to be faster and more nimble fingered. In fact, both groups were equally fast. The older typists had developed clever, timesaving strategies that involved fewer finger movements and reading ahead in the text, which made up for their slower reaction times.

Younger and older people matched on education, intelligence, health and other variables that may affect memory, show only minimal differences in learning ability, says Dr. Felicia Huppert of Addenbrooke's Hospital in Cambridge, England. When 80 adults aged 63 to 91 were given one German lesson a week for three months, more than half passed an examination at a level which schoolchildren normally reached after three years. The same group were taught to play the recorder and continued to play for pleasure long after the training was concluded.

Experience means that we can calculate when to cut corners without even thinking about it. We continually evaluate and refine. We also get to think in a process known as "chunking," which means we lump specialized knowledge together until it seems to be a single piece of information. The first few times you make an omelette or do a series of exercises you have to refer to instructions. With practice, you carry the whole thing in your head as a single operation. That's chunking.

And another thing—retired professionals, especially teachers and journalists, score higher in vocabulary tests than college students. Not surprising, given those years of reading, listening, viewing, talking, writing. Exercise the brain cells and they'll serve you well.

CARRY ON DRIVING

Professor Thomas Scott, who first got behind the wheel in 1924, passed the Institute of Advanced Motorists' test in 1993, when he was 86. In the same year, an 84-year-old woman passed her driving test, having been required to retake it after an accident, and—here's the bad news—a man of 82 drove south for 20 miles in the fast lane of a highway going north. Examples such as these suggest that there's no easy answer to age limits on safe driving. When researchers from the Duke University Center for the Study of Aging and Human Development looked into the effect of age on driving skills, and compared older and younger drivers, they found that healthy people aged 65-plus made fewer errors than those aged 18 to 19 or 25 to 35, and specific driving skills were judged either superior or unchanged. Greater caution and reluctance to drive in poor conditions are characteristic of older drivers. Crashes involving older people are thought to be due to lapses in concentration, difficulty in maneuvering, driving too slowly and failing to give way. No radios, no cassettes and no conversation with passengers is the advice given by some psychologists to older drivers in order to avoid distractions.

1. Do things your way, not the young way—and that means giving yourself time without pressure when doing, thinking and deciding.

2. Plan one project at a time, with minimal interruption—that's the way we work best as we get older and it's neither better nor worse than younger methods.

3. Retirement doesn't mean you stop thinking. Take up a new interest that exercises memory and requires reasoning power and problem-solving skills. This doesn't necessarily mean having to get bookish or academic. Dance classes as well as language courses can exercise memory; car maintenance or sewing your own clothes involves reasoning power and problem-solving skills. And remember, take on the learning slowly. You'll retain it longer.

4. Playing cards and doing crossword puzzles keep the mind sharpened.

5. New experiences, such as spending holidays in unfamiliar places, are stimulating. Read up on the history of a place before you go and write about the adventure when you get back.

6. Don't say all you want to do is hang around old friends. Get out and meet new people. Make an effort to get to know them.

7. If you have grandchildren, teach them new tricks. If you don't have grandchildren, borrow someone else's.

8. Don't be put off by new gadgetry and ever changing technology. You may take longer to master it than the average schoolchild, but you'll get there in time.

MAKING THE MEMORY WORK BETTER

Most people in middle age experience that irritating phenomenon of having a word or a name on the "tip of the tongue " but are unable to recall more than the first letter, if even that. Even a very familiar word or name. Suddenly it's gone, and equally suddenly it comes back. It's a case of memory getting slower, not necessarily less accurate. We take longer to remember the name of someone, but usually get it right in the end.

One explanation for this is that brain activity stops short of triggering all the necessary information for proper recall. We know instinctively that it's better to give up than to struggle with the memory, and when it comes through later, it's rather as if the final connections do get made and the right switches are pulled in due course.

What everyone who has experienced this kind of memory lapse in midlife wants to know but hardly dares ask is: Could this be the beginning of Alzheimer's disease? The answer is no. All the evidence suggests that Alzheimer's disease is different pathologically, psychologically and genetically. An article in the _British Medical Journal_ in 1992 called for new definitions for the memory impairment associated with age, and recommended new long-term research to help show what is normal for different older age groups. Age Associated Memory Impairment is now recognized as a distinct condition, with diagnosis mainly dependent on individuals themselves noticing their lapses and referring themselves to a doctor.

As things stand, we who begin to forget tend to take a gloomier view than is justified. True, there is a fairly rapid onset of name and face forgetfulness from the 50s onward, but names and faces fade in the memory of everyone after three to five years' absence of that person. True, we find it harder to retain unrelated facts, but so do younger people. That's why they make shopping lists, too.

Researchers now say that it is not so much that we forget more, as that we have more to remember. The older we get, the more information we have to store, but our powers of recall don't grow to meet the input. We remember incidents from our youth more clearly than recent events mainly because they had novelty value and still have great significance. A first sexual encounter, first love, job promotion or first holiday abroad are especially exciting and are memorable because they were an important part of our development.

Oldest memories also get repeated over the years, and the more we relive them the more permanent they become. Some researchers maintain that older adults are simply more economical with their memories. They eliminate recent trivial items such as what they had for lunch yesterday, simply because they've had lots of lunches and there's nothing to be gained from the memory of yesterday's meal unless it was especially significant.

A number composed of up to seven digits can be recalled immediately by people of all ages, but if more digits are involved, older people recall less well than younger. This brief, immediate recall uses short-term memory, and for the material to stick it has to be transferred to the more enduring long-term memory, which is thought to be a different brain function.

Older people appear to have difficulty in transferring items to long-term memory. However, failure to make the transfer can occur at any age. What was hard to remember in youth—for some people, dates and numbers for instance—becomes even harder to remember in later years. A great deal depends on what interests and what fires the imagination.

ALCOHOLIC EFFECTS

A common side effect of alcoholism is memory loss, but it may not be due to excessive loss of brain cells—a discovery that could be good news for those who can't stop overdrinking. Danish scientists Dr. Grethe Badsberg Jensen and Dr. Bente Pakkenberg of the Bartholin Institute studied the brains of long-term alcoholics who had died from their addiction. They found loss of connecting matter, but no loss of brain cells themselves, which suggests that memory could be re-established through treatment and prolonged abstinence. There's no evidence that moderate alcohol intake impairs brain power. On the contrary, one or two drinks a day can help preserve reasoning skills according to scientist Joe C. Christian of the Indiana University School of Medicine, whose evidence comes from comparing identical twins with different drinking habits.

Absentmindedness, something attributed to professors and, for some reason, women during menopause, is unlikely to have anything to do with aging. It is a hazard of skill and familiarity, which is why you might pick up a dishcloth rather than a knife when preparing potatoes, or put the tea kettle in the cupboard and begin to fill the cup from the tap. Such memory lapses occur when we're preoccupied with something else while taking the action. We might be thinking of the next job to be done, worrying about an impending exam, or wondering what to make for the evening meal while doing some other routine job. Such errors are known to affect both men and women regardless of age.

Loss of memory may be due to poor health, taking certain medicines or drugs, alcoholism, emotional stress or anxiety. People with high blood pressure have been found to have poor short-term memory; people with low blood pressure have also reported poor memory. Severe iron deficiency has been linked to memory disturbance. Lack of vitamin B_{12} in people over 60 may cause memory loss. Age itself is only one factor.

MEMORY EXERCISES

TO REMEMBER A NAME

- When you are being introduced, listen for the name and pay special attention to it.

- During conversation, try to use the name a few times.

- If you don't want to risk over-familiarity, say the name to yourself instead. Repetition helps, so if you have the chance, wait a few seconds and repeat it to yourself. Then repeat it two more times, each time leaving a longer gap between. The increasing pauses and four repeats force you to sustain attention and fix the name into long-term memory.

- Link the name to an image with a similar sound. Rhyming always makes things more memorable. It's easy with Mary, you can think of her feeding a canary, or being quite contrary.

- If rhymes don't appeal, try connecting the name with someone famous who has the same name.

- Connect a name with a face by linking it with some physical characteristic. Red Ted is easy for someone called Ted who conveniently happens to have red hair. Use any visual or verbal associations such as occupation, similar word, name of famous person, and always make a mental image.

TO REMEMBER NUMBERS

- Make meaningful patterns out of them. Supposing you want to remember that on May 16, 1998, it will be your friend's 45th wedding anniversary. You can try to make a pattern with 5, 16, 98, 45, using perhaps your house number and postal code, your children's ages, or any set of digits that you can recall easily. If you're stuck, try numbers matching months of the year, so that "5" is "May," etc. One example of an easy pattern: Mount Fujiyama is 12,365 feet high, which could become 12 months in the year and 365 days. How could you forget?

- The easiest way to recall a PIN number is to change it to correspond with the date and year of your birth, or that of a close relative. (But don't forget about security—choose something that isn't too easy to guess.) Alternatively, write the number down and work out a set of associations that can be recalled through a simple sentence. If you can't think of anything immediately,

EXERCISE AIDS MEMORY

After three months of regular exercise, women aged 55 to 75 not only gained in physical fitness, they also gained in short-term memory compared to a non-exercising group. All they did to increase their ability to remember a series of numbers when tested before and after was to walk three times a week for 20 minutes. Long-term memory did not, unfortunately, get a similar boost.

return to the numbers later, jotting down possibilities until you make a coherent and memorable pattern.

To REMEMBER A FACT OR WORD

- Similar sounds and rhythms can replace rhymes for remembrance. A way to remember that espresso coffee is black is to think of espresso blacko. Do you know which word is French for strawberry and which for raspberry? Think of the short straw—*fraises*, the shorter word, is for strawberries; *framboises* is raspberries. Concoct your own memory aid by using word association for an item that continually evades you.

- Make up a phrase or sentence which includes the words that you want to remember—it can be as nonsensical as you like. For instance, you might want to remember the name of a book after you've read a review or heard it talked about on television. The title of this book you are now reading could be remembered by "break the berry" and for my name, you can just "give thanks." Repeat your memory aide several times before consigning it to memory.

- Visual images always work better for some people. Think of the cover of this book or some other image that would remind you of its title. Repeat the title to yourself while visualizing the cover.

To REMEMBER WHAT YOU HAVE JUST READ

- After you've read a newspaper article or passage in a book that you particularly want to remember, follow the letters of the alphabet PQRST like this:

  P—**Preview** the passage quickly.

  Q—ask yourself **Questions** about the meaning of the item.

  R—**Read** it again, more slowly, trying to answer the questions.

  S—**Say** to yourself out loud what the item is about.

  T—**Test** yourself by answering the questions you tried earlier (you can practice this using a newspaper feature article).

- If you want to be able to recall a book or film, talk about the story to someone as soon as possible afterward. Write down a brief summary of the plot or tell the plot to someone a day or two later.

MEMORY TRAINING

Memory training may seem tedious, but it does genuinely exercise the brain—with good results. After 30 training sessions, elderly volunteers in one trial were able to remember a span of 40 or more digits. Give yourself time to do the memory exercises above. Take one at a time, create an example and try to recall it several times on the first day. Next day, add another exercise and a new example, recalling the previous one as well, and repeating it to yourself several times. Add on the rest gradually. Always ask yourself: "How can I remember this?" Then think of one of the methods you have learned and use it.

TO MEMORIZE LISTS

- For shopping lists, take a mental walk down the aisles of your supermarket or local shopping mall and try mentally placing each item you want to remember from the shelf or from the specific shop into your shopping cart.

- Make mental lists of unrelated objects by visualizing them around your living room. No need to put them in their legitimate places. The more bizarre your image, the more memorable it will be. Imagine, for instance, a birthday card tucked into the curtains, some spools of thread in a fruit bowl on top of the television, a camera or film pointing at the fruit bowl, rolls of fax paper piled up on the sofa. This could save you having to search in your bag or pocket for that creased piece of paper with the list written on it.

TO HELP YOU FIND THINGS YOU'VE LOST AND
TO STOP YOU FROM LOSING THEM IN THE FIRST PLACE

- Go back and take a second look in the place you first thought you'd left the object, searching more slowly this time, rather than continuing a search everywhere else.

- Keep things in regular places and if you choose somewhere new, stop for a moment and visualize the object in its new position.

- As you leave the house, check in your mind that you are taking everything you need. Do the same when you leave somewhere else.

- When out shopping, every now and then check the number of items you are carrying, especially when you've purchased another item and added another shopping bag.

EVERYONE USES MEMORY AIDS

A report in the *International Journal of Aging and Human Development* showed that commercial memory aids are an essential part of modern life, but not only for older people. Students and young adults starting a career use "hi-tech" aids like tape recorders and electronic memo pads. Many people use irons that shut off automatically or sound an alarm if left face down too long. Retired people use more bookmarks and favor plant alarms that are inserted into the soil and give a warning when a watering is needed. Alarm clocks, kitchen timers and diaries are commonly used by young and old alike. Life stage rather than age dictates the choice of memory aid.

TO RECALL MEMORIES OF THE PAST

- The time of year can trigger a memory, as can a color, fragrance, mood, season, poem, piece of music or particular outfit. Think about any of these references to set yourself on the path of further recall.

- Be observant. Notice the color, size, shape, texture and smell of something if you want to retain the memory of an incident or occasion for future reference.

HELPING THE MEMORY ALONG

- Make lists of things you plan to do and check each one off when you've completed the task.

- If you forget where you've put things, try to keep regular places for them and conscientiously return them to these places after use, every time.

- If you rearrange cupboards and put things in new places, write down a list of where they now go.

- To keep a clear head, check on your posture. There's a theory that a slumped neck and forward-jutting chin slow the flow of blood to the brain. Besides, a straight back and neck feel and look better.

- Relaxation helps improve memory. Before a lesson or lecture or anything you want to remember, take a few minutes to slow down the pace. Even if you don't have time to lie down for full relaxation, sit quietly, loosen shoulders and hold them back, and breathe evenly, listening to the ebb and flow of your breathing.

- Skipping breakfast can reduce mental alertness, and since there's a theory that fatty foods speed the processing of information, the old bacon-and-egg breakfast has its virtues, as well as its cholesterol-loading vices.

- Need to take medicines regularly? Use a kitchen timer as a reminder, or pin up notices with a list of the times in strategic places around your home.

NOT-SO-SMART DRUGS

Crossword puzzles may be better for the mind than bingo, but taking a pill to enhance short-term memory, boost concentration and creativity must surely be a lot easier. There are around 140 so-called "smart pills" being developed in the United States, some of them to alleviate Alzheimer's disease, some with the goal of maintaining energy levels. They represent a major investment for the drug industry, potential big business for the future. Some smart pills are used under medical supervision for conditions like Alzheimer's disease, Parkinson's disease and memory disorders in elderly people. What makes them of wider interest is that they are also available without a doctor's prescription to the public through mail order businesses.

The two big questions: Do they work? and Are they safe? Straight away we are into that nebulous area of would-be miracle cures and placebo effects. Business executives who can afford them and students who can't are said to be the main users, and there are many anecdotal stories of their effectiveness, ranging from rave reviews about their inducing instant clarity of thought and long-term memory to cautious claims that they provide "quiet" energy, usually after several months of use.

Which? Way to Health, a British consumer guide to food and health, asked Professor Steven Rose, an expert in neurobiology, to look at the claims and scientific evidence behind eight of the most widely available smart drugs and nutrients in the United Kingdom. With a back-up team of five experts he examined acetylcar litine, choline/inositol/lecithin, Fast Blast (which contains phenylalanine), hydergine, Memory Fuel (containing choline), piracetam, pyroglutamate and vasopressin. He concluded, "There's no justification for the claim that smart drugs can be of any therapeutic or 'memory-boosting' use to normal, unimpaired humans."

In the same report, Professor James L. McGaugh, director for the Center for the Neurobiology of Learning and Memory, University of California, said: "There are many drugs that enhance memory in laboratory animals but, as yet, none has been found sufficiently effective or safe to warrant use in treatment of memory disorders in humans."

Some of the drugs surveyed boost the neurotransmitter acetylcholine in the brain, but the report said that healthy brains have a surfeit of this anyway, and don't need any more. And there's no convincing evidence for the effectiveness of other drugs that increase oxygen or glucose to the brain, such as hydergin, or those that widen blood vessels, like vasopressin.

The report also pointed out that evidence for effectiveness is flimsy, based on poorly designed trials, with often exaggerated claims. Even the benefits for Alzheimer's disease sufferers is not consistent, with only some patients responding and only a temporary decrease in symptoms. We'd all have heard if there really was a sure cure.

Animal tests may be impressive, but they often involve large quantities of drugs injected directly into the brain, which wouldn't reflect what happens to humans taking them in small amounts in tablet form. Some of the drugs, in prescribed doses, cause side effects like nausea, vomiting, headache and sleep disturbance. While smart drugs have their uses for some specific disorders, to take them without medical supervision would be very unsmart indeed, is the report's conclusion.

Deprenyl was not included in the enquiry, but is worth singling out since it has been publicized as "the most potent anti-aging drug available to Americans." Its conventional use is as an antidepressant. It is also used to slow the progression of Parkinson's disease. It has also helped improve memory in Alzheimer's patients in clinical trials. However, the characteristic that is receiving the most attention is its ability to improve sexual vigor in rats.

NOT SMART, BUT INTERESTING

An extract from the world's oldest tree species, the ginkgo, is recognized as an aid to memory, dizziness, tinnitus (ringing in the ears) and headaches. Dutch researchers Jos Kleijnen and Paul Knipschild, in a paper in the *Lancet*, gave details of the extract's ability to help patients with "cerebral insufficiency" (which is more or less the same as Age Associated Memory Impairment), defined as difficulties with concentration and memory, absent-mindedness, confusion, lack of energy, tiredness, decreased physical performance, depressive mood, anxiety, dizziness, tinnitus and headache. Ginkgo is licensed in Germany, where it has been used for 20 years to treat such symptoms, and also in France, Italy, Portugal and Switzerland.

Forty separate trials show "clinically relevant" results, though there are questions outstanding about whether six weeks or three months of treatment are needed to see improvements, and how long after this the treatment should continue. It doesn't work for Alzheimer's disease. Its action is said to boost blood circulation, mop up free radicals and increase neurotransmitters, and according to Professor David Warburton, director of the Human Psychopharmacology Group at Reading University, it has better evidence for efficacy than the new smart drugs. "Use it like spectacles or a hearing aid," he says. Gingko can be bought at health food shops. Side effects are rare— headaches, dizziness or stomach upset in 7 out of 10,000 people.

Deprenyl increases the level of neurotransmitters (which, despite the *Which?* report, do decline with age according to most experts). One neurotransmitter involved is dopamine.

The evidence for Deprenyl's effect on healthy brains is anecdotal. In a summary published in *Longevity*, a magazine noted for its interest in youth-extension products for baby boomers, writer Bill Lawren could summon up no more than "It may be well worth discussing with your doctor as a potential sexual invigorator or even as a general anti-ager," a statement that promises very little.

This doesn't have to mean the end of the story. It could be just the beginning. What happens in rats is indicative of what happens in humans, otherwise scientists wouldn't be very interested in them. The pharmaceutical industry wouldn't be investing large sums of money without the belief that research will deliver something promising in due course. What is anecdotal today could well be scientifically proven the day after tomorrow, though determining whether it is safe may take even longer.

The pharmaceutical company Glaxo has been working on a drug to improve memory for several years, and is now following up on human trials, though the company insists that it is intended for those with Age Associated Memory Impairment and not for the healthy individual. Maybe one day we'll get safe, effective pills that can boost our intelligence, aid our concentration and improve our sex lives. But we need long-term studies before that day comes.

GET LESS STRESSED

It used to be simple: stressed individuals, typified by their chances of developing heart disease, had type A personalities. They were go-getting executives who didn't know how to wind down. Then it was the turn of bored middle managers who had no executive power and were at the mercy of their type A personality superiors. They, we were told, were even more stressed and subject to coronary problems. Now we hear that bus drivers, in Denmark if not elsewhere, are *less* likely to have heart attacks if they *hate* their job than if they enjoy it.

There is, for the moment, no answer to this seeming contradiction of received ideas. Perhaps the Danish bus drivers happened to be blessed with protective genes or exercised in their time off and ate an especially healthful diet.

Generally, research shows that you don't have to be an executive, a middle manager or a bus driver to experience stress and its negative effects on health. Hostility toward fellow human beings, long and bitter arguments between couples, divorce, caring for a partner who has Alzheimer's, even a belief in fatality due to predictions from birth signs can deplete the immune system so that there is greater vulnerability to physical infections or chronic diseases.

FATAL BELIEVERS

Chinese-Americans who believe in Chinese horoscopes are in danger of developing a negative attitude that can prove fatal. If they suffer from serious conditions like cancer, heart disease, diabetes or peptic ulcer, and their astrology readings show an ill-fated combination of their disease and birth year, they die significantly earlier than nonbelieving Americans. This finding, reported in the *Lancet*, suggests a degree of fatalism—if it's in the stars, then why fight it. A more positive approach would be to see the situation as a challenge and prolong survival by changing to a healthier lifestyle.

A recent report from Sweden confirms the theory that adverse life events influence the risk of middle-aged men dying prematurely, and the influence was seen to continue for seven years. Among 752 men aged 50, selected randomly from the population and followed up for seven years, those who had suffered job loss, financial trouble, legal prosecution, divorce or separation or illness of a family member had higher-than-normal mortality rates. More than one "event" increased the risk, as did social deprivation. Deaths were from heart disease, cancer, or alcohol-related. The one encouraging finding was that "for men with a high amount of emotional support there was no evidence of an effect of life events on mortality." Intimate friends or a happy home life appear to promote an emotional and physical resistance to stress.

SIGNS TO WATCH FOR

Stress isn't all bad. A little is exactly what's needed for concentration, cooperative behavior, problem-solving, concern for others and increasing energy. In some instances it can be life-saving. The important thing is to realize when stress is getting out of hand and to do something about it.

Stress can be recognized by various kinds of behavior and reactions. If some of these signs feel familiar and fairly regular, then it's time to make changes. Have you experienced any of the following signs of being too stressed:

- recurring anger, irritability, feelings of hostility or resentment
- feeling overburdened, out of control, trapped or unable to change
- panic reactions with fast, shallow breathing
- guilt, feelings of hopelessness, sadness
- trouble concentrating and difficulty in making decisions
- difficulty in "turning off"
- double-checking everything
- depending on tobacco, alcohol or drugs to help relaxation
- inability to sleep, disturbed sleep pattern

GET POSITIVE

A problem shared is a problem halved. If something is worrying you or you feel totally stressed, talk it over with a friend, family member or counselor. You may feel better for a few tears and a confession of sadness, loss or low self-esteem.

Exercise to unwind. Run around the block. Physical exercise aids relaxation and gives the mind a break from worries and preoccupations.

Check your priorities. Make a list of tasks to do, decide which are essential and which can be postponed. You don't have to be perfect or super-efficient. Accepting your limits gives you a sense of being in control.

Be adaptable. If you feel overburdened, don't moan or get resentful. Find practical solutions or delegate tasks to others.

Be curious, look for change and welcome challenges. If you approach change with an open mind, and take it in small doses, you will feel you are in charge.

Give up caffeine, and if you are still smoking or overdrinking, go and get professional help.

Try smiling and laughter. Even smiling without feeling happy inside can change your mood to a positive one. Laughing relaxes muscles, slows the heart and uses up potentially harmful adrenaline.

Relax. Now and again during the day, let go of any tension—let your jaw drop, lips part, shoulders roll back. Breathe deeply and evenly, watching your breath rise and fall. Better still, attend classes in relaxation, yoga or meditation. Even a few minutes of meditation a day can make a big difference in your mental outlook.

Slow down the pace. Deliberately walk, rather than run. Give yourself extra time to get places so you don't have to rush. Remind yourself to get off the treadmill.

Be good to yourself. Forgive your mistakes, allow yourself time off and take time out to listen to music, read and commune with nature.

HOW POSITIVE DO YOU FEEL?

You can check if you have a positive outlook by asking yourself a few questions about how life was for you in the last week. Psychologists in California use a test called PSOM, Positive States of Mind Scale, to check attitudes and life satisfaction. They ask questions like whether, in the last week, you managed to get on with jobs and tasks that needed to be done, without inner, as opposed to external, distraction. Were you able to try a new way to solve problems or express yourself creatively? Did you gain satisfaction from taking good care of yourself or someone else? Could you say you felt relaxed, without distractions or excessive tension? Were you able to enjoy bodily senses, intellectual activity and doing things you ordinarily like, such as listening to music, enjoying the outdoors or lounging in a hot bath? Were you able to commune with others in an empathetic, close way, as in talking, walking, going out, or just being in company? Too many negatives to these questions suggest you need a change in mental attitude and possibly expert help.

BEATING DEPRESSION

Midlife is not the biggest time for depression. Around one-quarter of women and one-eighth of men in Western society will suffer at least one episode of depression during their lifetimes. It can happen at any age, with women always more susceptible, but at menopause and during the postmenopausal decade, there is a fall in the prevalence of general psychiatric problems. Later life is the testing time when loss of a partner, chronic illness, isolation, loss of independence and poverty are more likely to occur. These events and circumstances can lead to depressive symptoms in some people, especially women, since they live longer than men. Even then, many experiencing difficult life events remain positive. Research shows that a good social network or intimate relationship is a great defense against depression.

Stressful events are not always the total cause. Around 15 percent of cases of clinical depression in older people are thought to be associated with biological factors. The biological mechanisms involve neurotransmitters, especially noradrenaline and serotonin, which may be depleted in people who get depressed. The newest investigations on causes of depression are focusing on brain peptides, chemicals that affect neurotransmitters and also trigger hormone activity.

People affected by biological factors may have bouts of depression throughout life. The predisposition can run in families, and there is almost certainly a genetic link, though by no means everyone with the particular genetic makeup gets depressed. A stressful environment may be the trigger.

When it comes to treating depression, antidepressants which reverse the low-serotonin effect, such as Prozac, are very effective and have fewer toxic side effects than the older tricyclic drugs. Not that these are without side effects—tiredness, insomnia, restlessness and even violent behavior have been reported. Despite the publicity for Prozac as a "happiness pill," its manufacturer, Eli Lilly, takes a more cautious line and sees it as a treatment for true depression rather than a popular cure-all.

Since depression seems to be a mix of biology and circumstance, psychotherapy may be part of the treatment, too. Medication along with some form of short-term psychotherapy is the combination recommended by the National Institute of Mental Health. In the United Kingdom, the Royal College of Psychiatrists' guidelines for older patients put the emphasis on antidepressants for severe depression followed by "anxiety management" techniques, which include counseling.

Are there ways to protect against depression in later life? Staying active and in touch with other people as we age seems to be the best defense, according to research. Talking, laughing and having a sense of curiosity all alleviate stress and depression. Having a pet or even a plant to look after may have a protective effect. If a partner dies, close friends and family members are needed for their support. Outside interests that

DOES DIET AFFECT THE MIND?

One thousand women and men aged 18 and over were asked to fill in questionnaires about their eating habits. They were also assessed for anxiety and depression to see what links there might be between diet and mental state. The key finding was that women who ate large quantities of fruit and vegetables had the most positive mental health compared to other women. There was no association between diet and mental health in men, and no significant statistical association with other foods. Do health-conscious women also have a positive mental outlook, or is there the possibility that diet itself influences mental heath? The researchers don't know. Nor can they say why fruit-and-veggie-eating men don't get the same benefit.

THE CAN-DO ATTITUDE
IS MORE IMPORTANT THAN BIRTHDAYS

Ronald Reagan was elected president at the age of 69. Wagner composed *Parsifal* at the same age. Freya Stark continued as an explorer and writer until she was in her 90s. Golda Meir became prime minister of Israel at the age of 70. Roget published his *Thesaurus* when 73. If you believe what you read in newspapers, here are a few more reminders of some things that older people can do. Two Taiwanese women aged 78 were arrested for prostitution, along with 50 others aged 60-plus who were making a living at it. Mrs. Margaret Anne Neve, who died at the age of 111 in 1903, was remembered walking to market regularly and wielding a light spade at the age of 108. And a certain Mr. Tom Brown was 83 when he floored an intruder aged 24. Mr. Brown had been a weightlifter and wrestler in his youth, and according to a newspaper report of the incident, he still exercised regularly.

---

have been developed are there to be taken up to reduce the sense of loneliness and isolation. Pre-retirement planning and careful management of pensions are some defenses against poverty. A determination to be in charge even with chronic illness can reduce loss of independence. And an awareness of the symptoms of depression can halt its progress if help is sought quickly.

NEGATIVE THINKING

- People who express life in negative terms or look to the future as doom laden have reduced immune systems. Psychologist Judith Rodin from Yale University led a team that studied the "explanatory style" of people aged 62 to 82 years, and then also measured their immune systems from blood samples. There was a clear link between the pessimists and a reduced immune system, making pessimism a possible psychological risk factor for a variety of physical diseases.

- If you are female, 40-plus and reached adolescence at a period of increasing opportunities for female achievements, you are more vulnerable to depression than if your adolescence was at a time of stable or decreasing opportunities for women. This odd finding comes from a report by B. Silverstein and D. Perlick of the City College of New York psychology department. A case of dashed hopes and promises turning sour, presumably.

- Research shows that many people dread old age well before they get to it. A survey of under-35-year-olds showed that 60 percent were definitely not looking forward to getting old. Most of them defined "old" as being in the mid-60s, though one in three thought it was nearer 50-something. Fear of age could be a growth industry. Panic at physical signs of aging, dread of diseases such as cancer, avoidance of younger people and embarrassment at going to social events and even restaurants much frequented by younger people are some of the phobic symptoms reported by therapists and health workers.

RECOGNIZING ACUTE DEPRESSION

After two weeks of the following, it is time to get help:

- feelings of worthlessness, emptiness or guilt
- impaired concentration, inability to make decisions
- loss of energy, boredom and fatigue
- thoughts of suicide
- appetite and/or sleep disturbance
- agitation, loss of memory
- complaints of vague aches and pains, headache, etc.

Low-key depression is less easy to define, though it is recognized and even has a name, dysthymia. It is long-term, chronic, with typically gray symptoms like low mood, fatigue, a general feeling of joylessness, but just sufficient energy to keep the sufferer going so that he or she is not fully aware of being in a depressed state.

Diagnosis may occur only when some event turns it into full-blown depression.

A GOOD NIGHT'S SLEEP

Do we need less sleep as we get older? Do older people suffer more from sleep problems than does the rest of the population?

Around 8 to 10 percent of adults under 30 say they often or always have sleep problems. The figures rise gradually with age, always with more women reporting regular sleep problems. (One theory for this is that women in middle age are still suffering, many years after, from a disrupted sleep pattern caused by the need to be alert to their crying babies, though another cause could be a hormone response to crying infants that begins after pregnancy and ever ends.)

By 70-plus, a good 29 percent of women and 20 percent of men complain of inadequate depth of sleep, frequent awakenings in the night and insufficient sleep.

When scientists have studied older people in sleep laboratories, they have observed "a reduction in sleep efficiency," meaning less REM (rapid eye movement) sleep associated with dreaming, reduced slow wave (restorative) sleep and an increased number of shifts from one stage of sleep to another. Men tend to experience more and longer wakenings. Women are more sensitive to noise. Daytime napping is more common among men, and in 25 percent of 70-year-olds, rising to 45 percent of 80-year-olds. Disturbed night sleep may be the cause of day napping, though lifestyle factors—from lack of stimulation to stuffy rooms—may also contribute.

Circadian rhythms alter with age, possibly to different degrees in men and women. Research has shown that body temperature and the secretion of the hormone melatonin are different in old and young people. Melatonin is secreted by the pineal gland in the brain during sleep and levels decline with age, affecting the sleep pattern and the response to light. These changes make older people susceptible to waking at unsocial hours. The body clock "awakes" an hour earlier in the morning with each decade from the age of 60.

Sleep patterns may alter with age, but individuals can be good or bad sleepers at any time of life, and the differences between individuals are greater than the differences between old and young.

Anxiety and worry over loss of sleep have a compounding effect. The worry itself can cause exhaustion and tension—which in turn interferes with sleep. We don't all need seven or eight hours a night and some individuals get by happily on less. Sometimes, talking over the problem with a doctor or counselor can help you sort out concerns over sleeplessness.

FIGHTING INSOMNIA

Mostly, insomniacs know when they are beaten, and may be tempted by the magic of a pill. Millions swallow their nightly tranquilizers and sleeping pills, often for many addictive years. Doctors now prefer to prescribe them for a short period only, perhaps three or four weeks.

THE BIG SNORE

About 20 percent of middle-aged people snore. A small percentage of them, about 2 to 4 percent, suffer from a potentially dangerous condition called sleep apnea. The main symptoms are loud snoring followed at intervals by a deep, snorting breath and an alarming (to any listener) moment of breath-holding silence before the pattern is repeated. This semi-awakens the sleeper, who may be regularly deprived of deep, refreshing sleep leaving him or her (statistically more often him) vulnerable to drowsiness even, for instance, when driving during the day. The uneven breathing also increases the chance of developing high blood pressure or having a stroke. Losing weight, removing the tonsils, remodeling the palate or wearing a special breathing mask may help. Mild and occasional snorers will benefit from sleeping on their sides, with ping-pong balls sewn into a pocket in the back of their pajamas to encourage them to stay that way. Special adhesive strips are also available that can be worn across the bridge of the nose to help reduce snoring. Other factors besides age itself can affect the quality of sleep. Physical illness that causes pain, joint stiffness or other discomforts, a weak bladder, respiratory ailments, depression and anxiety can all upset sleep patterns. Drugs such as beta blockers for high blood pressure, ephedrine for asthma or diuretics to decrease fluid retention and stimulate the passing of urine, may also disturb sleep.

MAKING UP ON LOST SLEEP

Is it a good idea to get a nap later in the day if you had to get up early or suffered a sleepless night? A midday nap can make it harder to get to sleep at night, and the ideal thing is to retire early the following evening to make up the lost sleep. But the body tends to slow down after lunch, which is how the siesta got started, and catching up occasionally at this time can prevent an exhausted evening. In hotter climates the afternoon siesta is a ritual. But a 15-minute nap may be more refreshing for many people than a longer, deeper sleep. A ten-minute relaxation period, spent sitting or lying down with eyes closed, is just as good.

There are many books and tapes on the market offering different ways to beat insomnia. Some advocate a strict routine even if it means tossing and turning in bed for hours. Others recommend going to bed only when tired. Give any method a few weeks before writing it off.

Keep a sleep diary for a week, recording when you go to bed, get to sleep and wake up. Also, note your state of mind, whether something is worrying you, making you angry, and interfering with your sleep. Doctors are now using sleep diaries to help find the best nondrug approach.

TEN NONDRUG WAYS TO HELP YOU SLEEP

1. Don't drink anything containing caffeine late in the evening, and that includes cola drinks as well as tea and coffee. Chamomile and other herbal teas are relaxing and soothing.

2. Milk- and malt-based drinks at night really do aid sleep. They contain a substance called tryptophan, which is converted in the brain to serotonin, a sleep-inducing chemical. Other foods containing tryptophan include eggs, cheese, turkey, nuts—not to be recommended for nightcaps but good for earlier in the evening.

3. Relax in a warm bath and wind down slowly before going to bed. Add a few drops of aromatherapy oils to the bath water. Pour a few more drops on your pillow.

4. Slow, gently rhythmic music may have a soporific effect on brain waves. Tapes playing sounds like waves beating on the shore or heartbeats are sold to get babies to sleep, and the same could apply to adults.

5. Reading in bed gets some people off to sleep, though it can have the opposite effect and keep you turning the pages until you finish. Choose a heavy rather than an easy read.

6. Try to go to bed at the same time every night, following a regular routine. Get up at the same time, too, and keep to the pattern if you can.

7. Try an herbal pillow. They often contain lavender or hops and are said to induce drowsiness.

8. Alcohol in small amounts may work, and a nightcap is worth a try. But keep it moderate—too much alcohol can mean a deep sleep followed by too much wakefulness a few hours later.

9. If you wake in the early hours, instead of tossing and turning, practice relaxation, paying special attention to facial muscles. Lie on your back with hands resting lightly on your abdomen, or on one side with knees bent in the classic relaxing position. Check your facial muscles from time to time to make sure you are still relaxed.

10. Earplugs and eyeshades may help if you are sensitive to surroundings. A sunny bedroom benefits from heavy curtains to keep the morning light out.

CHAPTER SIX

The Lifestyle Challenge

REAL-LIFE MIDLIFE—
BETTER THAN YOU THOUGHT

The publicist for the publishers had been having a hard time. She was trying to promote a popular book on osteoporosis, directed at women age 40-plus, and had encountered unexpected resistance. Some newspapers, she discovered, had a policy they defined as "no gray hairs." The color magazine supplements were particularly intractable. This was not because all their readers were young. It was, they explained, because the "grays" preferred to identify with younger people.

Women's magazines were equally adamant. "We don't want gray hairs on our pages," and "We don't want to seem 'old' even when addressing older women" were two remarks she encountered.

When "grays" do intrude on editorial pages, they get a very curious image. "Elderly pair tortured by sadistic raiders" ran one headline. How old was this pair? Both of them 65, according to the report, the age of many (mainly male) politicians, successful businesspeople, film stars, authors and television personalities.

In December 1993, a camera adver-
tisement was headlined, "This Christ-
mas, shoot Granny and put her in a
box." Just joking, with that extra lithe
touch of sexism for flavor. If you
don't like that one, you may warm to
this headline instead: "Fay Weldon, a
sexy rich granny having fun," which
leaves out "famous" but sums up
very well the things you have to be
in order not to be tainted by ageism,
and, for good measure, sexism.

> "Our parents' generation were
> ancient at our age, past it. We are
> more active, take greater care of
> ourselves. We're the 'new old,' but
> people don't make films about us."
>
> —Actor Jack Nicholson at
> 55 (The Independent,
> February 23, 1993)

"Mutton dressed as lamb," "old biddy," "hag," "crone," "witch"—these
are all excellent examples of the sexist side of ageism. And how about
"old fogy," "old codger," and even "dirty old man" for intensity and
dislike.

Older people are often featured as frail and dependent victims—like
that tortured couple above—or as some sort of joke when they show
they can drink, enjoy sex or have strong convictions just like everyone
else. Television comedy sitcoms, with one or two exceptions, depict
older people as crotchety, out of touch and *foolish*. Like Betty Friedan's
housewives before modern feminism, they are not to be taken seriously.

And we all laugh, pretending that we will never be old, will never be
disempowered, and will magically remain distanced from the inevita-
bility of aging.

The brainwashing starts early. When 11 year olds in Australia were
asked to draw pictures of old men and women, they drew people with
wheelchairs and walkers, slippers and aprons. The children reflected
the commonly held belief that aging is a degenerative biological process
that will inevitably lead to illness and breakdown, concluded the re-
searcher. They have received this idea from children's storybook illus-
trations, cartoons and comics, but not necessarily from the appearance
of their own grandparents who would probably be in the 60-to-75 age
range.

A survey of local government employers in the United Kingdom in 1993 exposed a series of stereotypic ideas when it came to hiring older people. "Over the hill and on the scrap heap at 50," "the brain deteriorates with age," "you don't get your money's worth from older people," were all typical attitudes. Despite equal opportunity employment and antidiscrimination policies, only about one-third of the employers, all involved in local government, included age in them. Unlike the United States, there is no legal constraint against age discrimination in the United Kingdom.

With ideas like these in circulation, many of them lumping together ignorance, prejudice and confusion about middle and old age, it is no wonder that headline writers, journalists, television filmmakers, advertisers and greeting card manufacturers (just take a look at greeting cards congratulating people on becoming grandparents) don't know how to depict anyone over 35 or don't want to be identified with anything that smacks of "the grays."

THE BEST TIME OF OUR LIFE

We are told that things are changing. Advertisers are now aware that people in midlife, some at any rate, have money to spend. They renovate their homes or buy new ones and decorate those instead. They go on vacations, place bets and don't get into debt. They buy toys for their grandchildren and anti-aging creams, have cosmetic surgery and get their hair done.

Not everyone is in this fortunate position in midlife, though. Loneliness, poverty, disability and bereavement paint a very different picture and every society needs built-in support systems, both political and personal. But these misfortunes are not specific to middle age. Consider the things that are:

- A mortgage, if there is one, may be close to being paid off.
- Experience and judgment replace the searchings and uncertainties of youth.
- Marriage, if it has survived, has fewer pressures than at any time previously—no small children to look after, plenty of freedom, companionship and independence.

- Adult children are likely to be settled and a source of pride and pleasure.
- Adult children, as they acquire their own families, tend to get closer to their parents.
- Grandchildren are usually sources of pleasure without too much of the responsibility.
- Friendships are often tried and true, long-term and satisfying.

This is real-life midlife, not just an aging process, but a positive experience in its own right.

In 1989, the MacArthur Foundation set up a seven-year research program focusing on middle age. It is known as MIDMAC, and the age range under scrutiny is from 30 to 64. One of the first observations from surveys was that the midlife crisis was the exception, not the rule. Younger people, nurtured on what MIDMAC director Gilbert Brim has called "widely shared cultural beliefs and untested theories about middle age," have got it totally wrong. While they have a picture of older people living in the past and worrying about money for health care, older subjects surveyed were talking about the stress of coping with a million current demands. They were having the busiest time of their lives.

Middle-aged people don't go in for great revelations borne out of emotional crises. They have transitions, gradual realizations that they need to slow down their pace or change their goals. More time for family life, a resolution to switch to a healthier lifestyle, an acceptance that they won't make it to the White House or even to their boss's position, or a desire to

GLORIA STEINEM

"For me, turning 50 felt like leaving something, but 60 feels like arriving in an exciting new country. You don't care about trying to look 30. I couldn't care less about sex, and that is wonderful. Your brain is free to think about other things. You're free from jealousy or competitiveness. I feel kind of peaceful about my body. I admire that it knows something I don't, which is how to age."—*Gloria Steinem at 60* (Longevity, July 1994).

pay something back to society in the form of volunteer or community work are all typical signposts of midlife found by MIDMAC researchers.

This does not necessarily mean the end of personal ambition, but it means coming to terms with realistic ambition. What people want most is to struggle and succeed, says Gilbert Brim. They seek a level of "just manageable" challenges.

The giving up of the dream, whether it's the brilliant career or the home with a swimming pool, is an enormous liberation according to Ronald Kessler, a MIDMAC research director. It releases a great deal of tension and energy. Dreams that run counter to reality waste energy. Those who cannot adjust to reality may well succumb to a midlife crisis, having spent a great deal of emotional energy deluding themselves until reality intervenes.

Midlife psychological crises are thought to happen to people with extra vulnerability to life's knocks. They probably had crises in their teens, 20s and 30s, too. Only 10 to 12 percent of Americans suffer a crisis in middle age, and it is usually associated with divorce, work problems or serious illness, any of which could have happened in earlier years and in fact happen to comparatively few in midlife.

Satisfaction in midlife is not confined to Americans. In 1993, the United Kingdom marketing organization Mintel found that people aged 45 to 54 were most likely, *of all age groups,* to say their lives were more satisfying now than when they were younger. And things are even getting better. Satisfaction levels were 5 percent higher than when Mintel did a similar survey in 1988. "Third agers" in the 55 to 64 age bracket were found to be demanding and knowledgeable consumers, requiring efficiency and impatient at any hint of being patronized.

In 1991, another survey on attitudes about aging reflected views of 626 people over 55 and 138 people over 75. It found that among those 55-plus, no less than 78 percent reported themselves to be in "very good" or "fairly good" health, and were enjoying the freedom of midlife. Seeing friends and family, traveling and going out, enjoying hobbies and pastimes and having a lot of contact with the younger generation all contributed to current happiness. Fewer financial problems were mentioned in 16 percent of cases, reflecting perhaps paid-up mortgages and freedom from business worries. Moreover, 44 percent of those surveyed expected to enjoy life more as they got older.

> *Sarah Bernhardt, the actress, suffered the amputation of one leg at the age of 71. She nevertheless continued her career, going on to play the lead in* Hamlet *on the Paris stage.*

They most probably will, too. A study of people from Dublin, Ireland, with an average age of 73, showed that their homes, social activities and religion were central concerns. Compared with a group aged on average 29, the older people were found to be less hard on themselves. They strived less and derived greater satisfaction from what they had achieved. They were no more bothered by health in terms of quality of life than younger people, though they reported more health problems.

There were some bad things to look forward to in later years. In one survey, financial difficulties were mentioned by 48 percent, loneliness by 20 percent and declining health by 36 percent—though among those over 75, only 6 percent claimed to be in "very poor health."

And the stereotypes have their effect. Those in midlife who don't have big spending power, and are not grudgingly admitted as semiretired members of the youth culture, get grayness with a vengeance. The older poor and disabled are still consumers, but they are offered gray walkers and wheelchairs, unsmart supportive armchairs and fewer choices and colors of products for basic needs. Compare this to the needs of the other economically inactive age group. Small children, learning to walk, get colorful objects suggesting fun and pleasure. We've got a long way to go.

SEX AND EXPECTATIONS

People with greater expectations for old age want to continue enjoying a sexually active lifestyle, goes current thinking. *The Janus Report*, published in 1993, which questioned nearly 3000 people aged 18 to 70, found that people in their 40s enjoyed more and better sex than when they were younger. Older people continued to have a regular sex life if they did so when they were younger.

Sociologist Alice Rossi, part of the MIDMAC team exploring development in the middle years, has found that women who start their sex lives early remain sexually active longer. Frequency of sex declines steeply with age, but levels of satisfaction change little over time.

We're talking mainly about people with sexual partners. Many older people live alone and do not have partners, sexual or otherwise. Some may express their needs by masturbating alone, while others by choice or circumstances live without sexual activity.

AGE IS NO PROTECTION

Elderly people can contract AIDS and other sexually transmitted diseases. The total number of AIDS cases in the U.S. of people over 60 jumped from 322 in 1981 to 1441 in 1992. The message is clear—you are never too old for safe sex.

And it depends on what you mean by sexual activity. Individuals differ but, from around 50, it normally takes longer for a man to achieve an erection. This is considered by some doctors to be due to changes in testosterone levels, but is more widely thought to be due to a diminished blood supply to the penis. It is normal for rigidity to be reduced, for ejaculation to be less powerful and for semen to be reduced. A rest period of around 24 hours or even several days may be needed before a repeat performance. On the other hand, it takes longer to ejaculate, which can be a good thing for partners. Some older men have no desire to ejaculate every time they have sex.

Women differ individually, but again there are typical physical changes. Lowered estrogen levels after menopause reduce blood supply to the vagina and nerves and glands surrounding it. As with men, sexual stimulation takes longer. The clitoris may be less sensitive. Orgasms may be shorter and less intense than they used to be. Thinning of tissue after menopause is associated with vaginal dryness and lack of lubrication, but many women continue to lubricate effectively even if it takes a little longer. Estrogen replacement therapy thickens tissue and restores lubrication. Water-soluble gels or estrogen creams also deal effectively with vaginal dryness.

Some women experience less interest in sex after menopause, and again estrogen replacement or the male hormone testosterone may help—the latter can produce other male sexual characteristics like deepened voice or body hair so it needs very careful monitoring. Other women find greater sexual freedom once past menopause when there is no need to use contraception.

The emphasis on performance and at being "good at sex" can be a kind of tyranny, an imposition of a culture of youth on older age groups. The important thing about sex is not how much you have or how much you "should" want, but how happy you and your partner are with whatever you're both getting. One of the advantages of growing older is being confident enough to free oneself from society's idea of what is right.

Some older couples have the confidence to explore new experiences now that there are no children around to interrupt privacy. Retirement, too, allows more time for sex. But others might prefer caressing to coitus, with the greater privacy afforded once the house is free of children. Gentle sensual pleasure can be as enriching for some as intense passion, perhaps more so when it is imbued with love and understanding. Orgasm may be the conventionally recognized aim, but there's no need to take it seriously.

If you do and it isn't happening, then this is the time for some honest talk—no blaming, no retreats from personal responsibility, just a shared acknowledgment and maybe a decision to get counseling or read some books on the subject. Some men hate the idea of a little help from their partner, and they need to find out why. Some women can't ask for more time or tell a partner what they want. Some older men and women find they have homosexual tendencies but feel they have to repress them. These responses have more to do with upbringing and attitudes than with age.

There are people in their 80s and 90s who continue to enjoy sex, though there can be a lot of people around to spoil the fun. Grown-up children (those in midlife) may be shocked, horrified or embarrassed. Nurses or staff in residential homes may feel it is their duty to protect elderly people from themselves, regarding sexual interest between residents as a sign of dementia. In a reversal of old-style morality, elderly lovers may have to keep their sex lives a secret.

GEORGE MELLY

Jazz singer, writer and art critic George Melly, at 68, recounts: "I am not able to drink as much as I used to—mainly due to an ulcer. I still get through several of what the medical profession insist on calling 'units'—with ice and lemon—a day. This lessening of my alcoholic intake, coinciding with my libido leaving the stage has left me, at night, with the happy sensation of having been unchained from a lunatic."

NOT ALL IN THE MIND

One British poll found that nearly one-third of men over 50 no longer have sexual relations, even though 23 percent of those in the survey had a partner. The reason was linked to anxiety triggered by medical problems. Fear of failure has long been understood as a reason for impotence in men, but more important is what has happened to cause the "failure" in the first place. Often that cause is physical. High blood pressure, diabetes and prostate problems are connected with narrowing of the arteries or damage to the nerve supply, both of which affect "performance."

Certain drugs, which may be used to treat the above-mentioned conditions, can in themselves cause impotence. Some medications used to treat high blood pressure, as well as certain antidepressants, antipsychotics, antihistamines, sedatives and tranquilizers are implicated, and a switch, under medical supervision, may help.

As mentioned earlier, low levels of the hormone testosterone could be the problem. An underactive thyroid is another possible cause of low libido. Lack of interest in sexual activity may be due simply to waning ability. An investigation of sexual activity among married men aged 70-plus, who were followed up five years later, suggested that reduced ability was a more likely reason for ceasing coital activity than psychiatric factors alone or combined with heavy drinking or smoking.

Treatment for underlying medical conditions may improve the situation but doctors have other ways to help treat impotence which are effective, though a trifle off-putting to anyone less than determined. Ask your doctor about special vacuum devices that can be used to constrict the shaft and trap the blood supply, creating an erection. Penile self-injection is another way to treat erectile problems and is available by prescription. A penile implant can create an erection via a pump action. All of these therapies have possible side effects, so be sure to discuss your options with your health care practitioner. Hormone treatment with testosterone, sometimes combined with other drugs, can be highly successful in treating impotence. The hopes for the future are drugs taken by mouth or absorbed through the skin in the form of creams or gels that will act immediately to dilate blood vessels. One skin treatment based on the drug minoxidil is expected to be going for FDA approval in the future.

LACK OF LIBIDO AND WAYS TO RESTORE INTEREST

- If you are taking drugs for any medical condition, check with your doctor for any possible effect on libido. Try to take medication at least an hour before planned sexual intercourse.

- Exercising regularly boosts sex hormones and helps the body to remain supple.

- Relax—try massage, meditation or simple relaxation exercises to cut down anxiety and stress levels.

- Alcohol, in moderation, can lower inhibitions though in greater quantities it may adversely affect performance.

- To help boost testosterone, take vitamin B_6 and zinc, both of which help synthesize male hormones.

- Try a side-to-side position or other variations to reduce pressure on stiff joints.

- A warm bath before sex is relaxing and reduces body stiffness. And there are those cold baths, reported earlier, which are said to restore interest.

MARRIAGE SECRETS

Having someone you like as a partner, a sense of humor, consensus on matters such as aims and goals in life, friends and decision-making skills—these are the ingredients for a good marriage according to 100 couples who had been together for 45 years or more.

Are arguments good for marriage? It depends on the way they are handled. Frustrating arguments, where women talk fast and men talk loud, speed up the heart rate and may lead to raised blood pressure and a negative effect on the immune system. Suppressed anger, however, is the fastest route to divorce.

Here are some ground rules for mature disagreements:

- Recognize when your arguments have a ring of the familiar, and decide which issues are worth fighting over.
- Listen with respect to the other person, even if you disagree.
- Make allowances for your partner's more irritating limitations and acknowledge that you might have some, too.
- Fight fair without being nasty.
- Laugh together afterward.

EMPOWERED RETIREMENT

More and more people are taking early retirement. The secret of making it work is to plan for it. Millions do by joining AARP, the American Association of Retired Persons. What this and other organizations representing older age groups offer is power through knowledge. And it's not only knowledge about insurance, pensions or health care coverage, it's also about political awareness.

Older people have paid a lifetime of taxes and continue to pay tax on pensions, income from savings and investments in retirement. When younger members of society are concerned about the cost of caring for older people, they need to be reminded of this. When politicians appeal for the old to give way to the young, they need to be made aware that both public and private sector employers must be responsible for old age as well as individuals. The Gray Panthers got the message decades ago.

ON GOLDEN POND

"The retired musicians of one of America's great symphony orchestras were interviewed. Their careers, which began in the 1930s and 1940s, were long, with retirement sometimes occurring when they were well over 70 years old. Older players were valued for their excellence and experience and were difficult to replace. Obsolescence was not a problem, and the gradual deterioration of playing with age was generally compatible with working to an advanced age. . . . The players liked their careers and usually cited artistic reasons and the current reputation of the orchestra for their satisfaction. Although the musicians continue to love music and listen to it after retirement, few continue to play seriously."

Summary of a paper entitled "The Great Symphony Orchestra—A Relatively Good Place To Grow Old In," which was published in 1988.

Retirement, we are now frequently told, is a comparatively new invention, a product of the early 20th century which may have made sense when many were employed in heavy manual work but now smacks of age discrimination. Today, when many people opt to retire early, while others clearly want and could continue long past the official age, there is growing awareness that the ideal is flexible retirement according to individual health or other situations. Even the idea of pensions is up for debate, with a minimum wage through life being discussed as a viable alternative. Now that we see that no job is for life, and rapid changes in technology make retraining a regular necessity, all age groups, including midlife, should have access to new opportunities.

Issues pinpointed by special interest groups include the following:

- When retirement nears, offers of part-time work alternatives, introduction to volunteering and training for working in groups should be made widely available.

- Recognition and sharing of past skills should be encouraged.

- Self-defense training could change the image of the old as victims and give them back the freedom to go out after dark.

- Men-only cooking classes and women-only financial management courses could redress the imbalance of a lifetime's earlier experiences.

KEEPING UP THE ASSERTIVENESS LEVELS

- You may have traditional skills like knitting, woodworking or gardening—use them to teach younger age groups, or join groups that barter skills and expertise instead of money.

- You may have been in the wrong job all your life. Now's your chance to explore things you like doing. Is it helping people, working with numbers, constructing or mending things, writing, singing or making music? Some of these interests have earning potential, others could lead to a new world of ideas, and friendships, through classes. There's more to volunteering than fundraising. Learn and use counseling skills in community self-help organizations. Join a group that shares your concern about a particular cause and get into local politics.

- Look for retirement projects that need professional help and offer your expertise.

- You can retrain and learn new skills at any age through local classes or distance learning. Learning is not only for profit, but enjoyment. It expands the mind and lifts the spirit.

- Knowledge is power. Get the information you need by joining national and local organizations for older people. Remember nothing happens unless you go out and get it.

- Join the computer age and go online to connect with others, especially if your are housebound.

TIME FOR CHANGE

- **Vacation tour packages** for 60-plus age groups cover a great deal of ground. It's not only cruising or coach tours nowadays. Skiing, walking, sailing, camping, painting, learning-to-swim, car maintenance—you have a choice. Benefits for members of the American Association of Retired Persons (AARP) include travel discounts with a number of firms.

- **Moving to a smaller home** may make sense financially, but too small could be a mistake. New hobbies and interests can make his and her workrooms or studies a very nice way to use up spare bedrooms. And when children and grandchildren come to stay, there's still space for them.

- **Home alone** can mean a sense of isolation. Retirement communities for active people of 55-plus offer security, varied types of housing and facilities like swimming pools and residents' restaurants. These may be the answer.

THE SECRETS OF HAPPINESS

What makes for successful aging and happiness in midlife? Social psychologists tend to fudge the answer by telling us that it all depends on "subjective well-being," meaning that you're happy if you achieve whatever you perceive as happiness-making. Increasingly, we can expect equally unsatisfactory gene-based answers, which tell us that some are born with more lugubrious temperaments than others.

Those who get their answers from surveys come up with everything you would expect. No, of course happiness does not come from success, fame, youth, good looks or wealth, even though in our weaker moments we tend to believe it does. The winner is always relationships and happy marriage and, if you have it, religious faith.

Relationships, when they work, are havens we trust, through long experience and feedback. They are places in which we can share negative feelings about ourselves, and a negative feeling shared is a negative feeling halved—much better than burying it as a shameful secret. Relationships are also places where we can laugh and let our fantasies and vulnerabilities show. Most significantly, relationships are where we can practice reciprocity.

"People who felt that their interpersonal relationships across the life course have been reciprocal—that they have both given to and received from others—will be the most successful in coping with the problems related to individual aging." So say social psychologists Toni Antonucci and James Jackson of the Institute for Social Research at Ann Arbor, Michigan. They suggest that reciprocity feels good because it avoids exploitation and implies a long-term trust, a conclusion few would argue with.

A sense of mastery and being in control of one's life is Margaret Hellie Huyck's explanation for happiness in midlife. She looked at areas of emotional investment and personal satisfaction, investigating two groups of 50 men, one aged 43 to 56, and the other aged 57 to 76, and two groups of 64 women, one aged 43 to 53, and the other 54 to 69.

Predictably, there was a shift from investment in work among the younger men to reduced investment in work and greater investment in marriage among the older men. Older men who were happy with this shift felt they had at least as great a sense of control as younger work-investing men.

A sense of success as parents was more important than work for the younger women. Far from regretting the empty nest, many of the older women talked of their sense of control over their leisure time, now that their children were self-sufficient. They called it "their time," when they could pursue "earned" freedom after having been conscientious wives, mothers and citizens.

Attitudes to health were different in the two female age groups. Many of the younger women assumed responsibility for their own health care and insisted they would not suffer the kind of physical frailties their mothers had taken for granted. They were heavily involved in exercising and healthy living. Those who did not invest in this way saw the lack as a personal failure or inability to organize their lives adequately. Such enthusiastic belief in self-care was absent from the older women, who tended to passively congratulate themselves on having few health problems "at my age."

THE WISDOM CRITERIA

Being wise is something we associate with age. But what does it mean exactly? Paul Bates, a MIDMAC fellow, says it includes factual and procedural knowledge, the capacity to cope with uncertainty, and the ability to frame an event in its larger context. The highest grades of wisdom occur around the age of 60. Modulation and balance are crucial elements; open-mindedness and tolerance are essential.

Deepak Chopra, author of *Ageless Body, Timeless Mind*, promotes meditation and relaxation as key steps toward wisdom, which he sees as inner harmony and liberation from the need to seek approval or to be judgmental or over-certain. "Forgiveness" is a contribution from Gail Sheehy as part of the wisdom to be achieved in midlife. Forgiving one's parents, society and the world, and acceptance of personal responsibility are part of wisdom's healing processes.

Betty Friedan's recipe for happiness is also concerned with autonomy and being in control of our bodies and our lives. In her book *The Fountain of Age* she talks of the importance of intimacy, entailing sharing of the "truth-telling authentic self" that emerges with time, and of finding the confidence to develop beyond the values of youth and stereotypical roles that separate the sexes.

The secret of happiness as we age is to see it as a new country to be explored. We can have greater confidence and self-knowledge than ever before. We can be more resilient and less bothered by what other people think—even the ones who think ageist—and we can have the time of our lives.

SEVEN MYTHS ABOUT AGING EXPLODED

1. Living alone

Not everyone is a Sun City seeker. Some older people like to be alone, seeking out a social scene in small doses. More than one-third of Americans over 55 live alone and like it, says the American Association of Retired Persons. They like neighborhoods with a mixture of age groups, though a growing number prefer living in an apartment block with other older persons.

A survey of New Yorkers aged 60-plus, from the New York Center for Policy on Aging, found that they kept close to home using their own neighborhood "villages"—local shops, banks, pharmacies, churches and synagogues. Their main confidantes were relatives rather than friends, but many had friends living in the same block or nearby. Around 88 percent said fear of crime had little effect on whether they went out alone in the day. But 65 percent feared going out alone at night.

2. You have to be rich to be healthy

People in higher income groups stay healthier and live longer, but money itself isn't the reason why. Yes, the rich can buy more and possibly better medical care, and if too lazy to exercise on their own can even employ a personal fitness trainer to keep them going. But money itself doesn't buy the healthy lifestyle—exercise, good eating habits, moderate alcohol intake, no smoking. It's the feeling of having greater control over one's life and keeping stress levels at bay that counts.

3. Older workers are over the hill

Older workers tend to have fewer accidents, less absenteeism, and greater output and job stability than their younger counterparts. In dis-

---

JUST GOOD FRIENDS

Patterns of friendship differ among women and men. In a summary of the differences, quoted in *Gender and Later Life*, men are reported as having fewer friends with whom to share troubles and joys, anxieties and hopes. An older man's best friend is often his wife, and work-based friendships are weakened at retirement. Women continue the support system with other women that they developed in earlier years and also develop closer ties of friendship with siblings. With increasing age, they tend to be visited more by friends than men do, but older men get out more in the evenings.

tance learning, the 60-to-65 age group gets better results than any other. Ample evidence shows that there is no sharp decline in mental ability with age, and the capacity to learn new skills and acquire knowledge and new attitudes is clearly present in middle age and beyond.

4. Old age means dependence

Only 5 percent of people aged 60 to 69 are unable to go out of doors alone. At 84-plus, 69 percent have no problem with stairs and over 90 percent lead independent lives in their own homes.

5. Old age means poverty

According to the American Association of Retired Persons, poverty levels do *not* increase for people over 65. In addition, older households—those headed by persons over 65 years of age—are less likely to receive public assistance than younger households. In fact, the median net worth of older households is over twice that of the U.S. average of $37,600.

6. Health and welfare spending on the elderly will be an enormous burden

Those over 85 consume a higher proportion of spending than any other age group, but they represent only a very small proportion of the population. Forecasts on future spending do not present a horror story. Although there will be an increased demand on resources as the elderly population expands, that increase is small until after the year 2011, when the Baby Boom generation hits retirement age, and even after that will be no more than 12 percent higher than present levels, says a report by J. Ermisch from the Joseph Rowntree Foundation.

7. There was once a golden age when being old was venerated

Satirical or unsympathetic images of old age are found in ancient Hebraic culture, early Christian and Greco-Roman writings and medieval literature—along with exhortations to respect and protect the elderly. Neither a past golden age nor universal denigration existed, though some societies valued their older citizens for their wisdom, experience or economic usefulness.

BREAKING THE AGE BARRIER

As this book has demonstrated, the way we get older depends on attitude and genes, a mix of free will and luck. The balance between the two never ceases to be important.

My mother, at 93, was sprightly, active, quick on her feet. A year later, the cartilage in one knee had completely worn out—from walking all her life (my parents never owned a car). She resisted using a cane at first, and grumbled that she was once a strong woman and look at her now. But she has adjusted and meets the challenges. She gets out mostly when escorted to visit her grand- and great-grandchildren, though if the weather is fine she struggles down the steps from her apartment alone for a short walk along the street, and then struggles even more to get up the steps home again. She has handed over most of the cooking to my father, a year her junior, but remains in charge. She faithfully does the exercises suggested by the physiotherapist, and gets her hair tinted honey blonde and always asks for new clothes for her birthday.

She is not, as she says, the woman she was, and we both know that there may be more difficult times ahead. We live a precarious balance between the acceptable present and a more difficult future. We live, inevitably, with impending death. This is true for all of us as we reach middle age and look into our own futures.

Acceptance and fight, acknowledgment and resistance—throughout our lives we continue to be offered these choices. For some, the fight may seem undignified, even neurotic—why resist the inevitable, why not give in to it with gentle acceptance? Whatever we do we won't live forever. For others, the fight offers true dignity and empowerment and its critics sound like defeatist wimps.

We need to remember our mortality and to find ways to come to terms with it. But as long as we live we can choose to live positively. It is possible to grow older gracefully and realistically, but with a kind of toughness, too.

Helen Franks, 1996

THE BIRTHDAY CHECKLIST

If you've made it this far through this book, you should be convinced that you can influence the way you are getting older, both in body and in mind. You will, perhaps, have decided to exercise more and review your eating habits. You can also keep tabs on how you're doing by comparing physical and mental ability, agility and attitude from year to year, and more specifically from birthday to birthday. On your next birthday, get hold of a sheet of paper, write down the answers to the questions below, and keep it tucked in the back of this book for reference and comparison at the end of the following 12 months.

PHYSICAL CHECK

1. How many hours a week do you exercise? Remember, it should be about 20 minutes of aerobic activity, involving brisk walking or running or jogging, for three sessions a week, plus warm-up and stretching exercises. Reread Chapter Three.

2. Check your pulse rate—details on page 19.

3. Run up a flight of stairs and check whether you get slightly, fairly or uncomfortably out of breath. Write down the result and try with the same stairs if possible in future years.

4. Are you as agile as you were? Can you stretch to touch your toes to the same extent as last year?

5. Are you as upright? Stand against a wall and if possible observe yourself in a mirror. Can you stand straight so that heels, hips, shoulders and the back of your head touch the wall behind you? (Don't cheat by hollowing your back or sticking your chin out.)

NUTRITION CHECK

6. Does your daily diet include at least three helpings of fresh vegetables and two to four pieces of fruit?

7. Do you eat fish at least twice a week, have sufficient fiber and calcium and keep fat intake low? See page 72 for Twelve Golden Rules on eating and drinking.

8. If your regular diet is less than ideal, do you get sufficient nutrients from vitamin and mineral supplements?

BASIC HEALTH

9. Do you have regular screening checks? When was your last screening for cancer, cholesterol, blood pressure, etc., and your last dental and eye exams?

10. Do you take more/less medication than you did last year?

11. Are you drinking too much, still smoking, eating a high-fat diet and getting little or no exercise? If the answer is yes, then now's the time to make the necessary changes for a less aging lifestyle and hopefully a different response next year.

MENTAL STATE

12. How many organizations/classes/groups do you belong to that involve regularly being with other people?

13. How many days a week do you join in a discussion, do crossword puzzles, practice a foreign language, read a challenging book or newspaper, or engage in some other mentally stimulating activity?

14. Is your outlook positive most of the time, or do you get discouraged by striving too hard?

15. Do you talk to someone when you feel discouraged or depressed?

16. Do you practice some form of relaxation when you feel stressed?

17. Do you aim for knowledge and harmony rather than approval?

18. Can you agree with the following statement? "I can live more healthily, I can take care of my body and my mind, I can feel optimistic about the future."

Bibliography

INTRODUCTION

"The Aging of the Human Species." Olshansky, S.J. et al. *Scientific American*, Apr. 1993.

The Health of Elderly People. HMSO 1992 (quoting Gothenberg report).

"Healthy Ageing: A Population Approach." Khaw, K. *Geriatric Medicine*, Mar. 1991.

Life Extension Report on Biomarkers. American Academy of Anti-Aging Medicine, Nov. 1993.

"Longevity: A Review of the Epidemiological Evidence." Palmore, E. B.

Physical Activity, Aging and Sports, vol. 1, ed. Harris, R. and Harris, S. Center for the Study of Aging, Albany, NY.

THE FITNESS CHALLENGE

Allied Dunbar National Fitness Survey, Sports Council and HEA, 1992.

"Are the National Fitness Survey Strength and Power Thresholds for Performance of Everyday Tasks Too High?" Skelton, D. and Young, A. Human, Performance Group extracts, Royal Free Hospital School of Medicine, London.

Bone Boosters. Moran, D. and Franks, H. Boxtree, 1993.

"Carnegie Inquiry into the Third Age." Evans, J.G. et al. Research paper no. 9, Carnegie Trust, 1992.

"Customary Physical Activity, Psychological Well-Being and Successful Aging." Morgan, K. et al., *Aging and Society*, vol. 11, 1991, pp. 399–415.

"Development in Health Status of a Group of Retired Subjects in Paris Region According to Their Practice of Physical Activity." Cassou, B. et al. *Revue de l'Epidemiologie et de Santé, Publique*, vol. 40, no. 5, 1992.

Devon/Senegal study, Faculte des Sciences, University de Cheikh Anta Diop, Dakar, Inserim Unit 1 Paris, *British Medical Journal*, vol. 306, Apr. 10, 1993.

Exercise and the Heart. Hardman, A. Report of the British Heart Foundation Symposium, 1991.

"Exercise Benefit." *Geriatric Medicine*, May 1992.

"Falls, Elderly Women and the Cold." Campbell, A.J. et al. *Gerontology*, vol. 34, 1988, pp. 205–8.

"Group vs. Home-Based Exercise Training in Healthy Older Men and Women, A Community Based Clinical Trial." King, A.C. et al. *Journal of the American Medical Association*, vol. 266, no. 11, Sept. 1991, pp. 1535–42.

"High-Intensity Strength Training of Nonagenarians." Fiatarone, M.A. et al. *Journal of the American Medical Association*, vol. 263, 1990, pp. 3029–34.

In Search of the Secrets of Aging. National Institute on Aging Department of Health and Human Services, May 1993, National Institutes of Health pub. no. 93-2756.

"In Shape." Reich, H. *Longevity*, Sept. 1993.

"Maximum Statistic Respiratory Pressures in Healthy Elderly Human Beings." McConnell, A. and Copestake, A.J. *Journal of Physiology*, vol. 467, p. 28, 1993.

Mobilistics Survey. *Active Life*, Sept. 1992.

"Physical Activity, All-Cause Mortality and Longevity of College Alumni." Paffenbarger, R.S. et al. *New England Journal of Medicine*, vol. 314, pp. 605–13.

"Physical Activity and Stroke in British Middle-Aged Men." Wannamethee, G. and Shaper, E.G. *British Medical Journal*, vol. 304, Mar. 7, 1992.

"Randomised Controlled Trial of Exercise in the Elderly." McMurdo, M.E. et al. *Gerontology*, vol. 38, no. 5, 1922, pp. 242–48.

"A Screening and Counselling Program for Prevention of Osteoporosis." Gutin, B. et al. *Osteoporosis International*, vol. 2, no. 5, Sept. 1992, pp. 252–56.

"Skeletal Muscle Weakness and Fatigue in Old Age: Underlying Mechanisms." Faulkner, J.A. et al. *Annual Review of Gerontology & Geriatrics*, ed. Cristofalo and Lawton, Springer Publishing, NY, 1990.

"Survival of the Fittest." Fishman, S. *Health*, May/June 1993.

"The Tennis Advantage." Higdon, D. *Longevity*, July 1993.

"Thermal Regulation and Hydration Levels in Aging." O'Reilly, K. *Physical Activity, Aging and Sports*, vol. 1, ed. Harris, R. and Harris, S. Center for the Study of Aging, Albany, NY.

"Who Exercises? Predicting Exercise in Late Midlife." Schnurr, P. et al. *International Journal of Aging and Human Development*, vol. 30, no. 20, 1990, pp. 153–60.

"Why Patients Consult and What Happens When They Do." Martin, E. et al. *British Medical Journal*, vol. 303, Aug. 3, 1991.

THE NUTRITION CHALLENGE

"Alcohol Abstainers, A Low-Risk Group for Cancer." Kjaerheim, K. et al. *The Globe*, Journal of the Institute of Alcohol Studies, July 1993.

"Alcohol and Ageing." James, O. Research Into Ageing briefing, Sept. 1992.

"Alcohol Consumption and Risk of Coronary Heart Disease." Jackson, R. et al. *British Medical Journal*, vol. 303, July 27, 1991.

"Alcohol Consumption by Elderly People: A General Practice Survey." Iliffe, S. et al. *Age and Ageing*, vol. 20, 1991, pp. 120–33.

"Asthma Linked to How Much Salt We Eat." *Which? Way to Health*, Oct. 1993.

Beat Sugar Craving. Stewart, M. Vermilion, 1992.

"Bone Density Parathyroid Hormone and 25-Hydroxyvitamin D Concentrations in Middle Aged Women." Khaw, K. et al. *British Medical Journal*, vol. 305, Aug. 1, 1992.

Britain's Flight from Alcohol, the Reality of Non-Drinking in the 1990s. Ansvar Insurance Company Ltd., Dec. 1992.

"Caffeinated and Decaffeinated Coffee Effects on Plasma Lipoprotein Cholesterol, Apolipoproteins and Lipase Activity." Superko, R. et al. *American Journal of Clinical Nutrition*, vol. 54, 1991, pp. 599–600.

"Calorie Restriction Diets Can Prolong Active Life." Kyriazis, M. *Geriatric Medicine*, June 1992.

"Cancer, Nutrition as a Cure." Goodman, S. and McTaggart, L. *What Doctors Don't Tell You*, vol. 4, no. 7.

"A Case-Control Study of Diet and Rectal Cancer in Western New Yorkers." Freudenham, J.L. et al. *American Journal of Epidemiology*, vol. 131, pp. 612–24.

"Cataract—What is the Role of Nutrition in Lens Health?" Bunce, E. and Hess, J. *Nutrition Today*, vol. 23, 1988, pp. 6–12.

"The Cholesterol Myth." *What Doctors Don't Tell You*, vol. 3, no. 1.

"Choosing Fats and Oils." *Which? Consumer Guide*, Oct. 1993.

"Coffee and Coronary Heart Disease." Myers, M. and Basinski, A. *Archives of International Medicine*, vol. 152, Sept. 1992, pp. 1767–72.

"Coffee-Associated Osteoporosis Offset by Daily Milk Consumption." Barrett-Connor, E. et al. *Journal of the American Medical Association*, vol. 271, no. 4, Jan. 26, 1994.

"Coffee, Caffeine and Cardiovascular Disease in Men." Grobbee et al. *New England Journal of Medicine*, vol. 323, no. 15, Oct. 11, 1990, pp. 1026–32.

A Comparison of Ten Selenium Supplementation Products. Clausen, J. and Nielsen, S.A. University of Roskilde, Denmark.

"A Controlled Trial of the Effect of Calcium Supplementation on Bone Density in Postmenopausal Women." Dawson-Hughes, B. et al. *New England Journal of Medicine*, vol. 323, 1990, pp. 878–83.

Dietary and Nutritional Survey of British Adults, OPCS HMSO, 1990.

"Dietary Fibre, Chemical and Biological Aspects." Southgate, D. et al. *Royal Society of Chemistry*, no. 83, 1990.

"A Dietary Key to Uncovering the Aging Process." Masoro, E.J. *NIPS*, vol. 7, Aug. 1992.

"Eat Walnuts for Your Heart." *Which? Way to Health*, Aug. 1992.

"The Effect of Dietary Supplementation with Vitamins A, C and E on Gall Mediated Immune Function in Elderly in Long-Stay Patients." Penn, N.D. at al. *Age and Ageing*, vol. 20, 1991, pp. 169–74.

"Effect of Vitamin and Trace Element Supplements on Immune Responses and Infection in Elderly Subjects." Chandra, R.K. *Lancet*, vol. 340, 1992, pp. 1124–27.

"Effect of Vitamin E and Beta Carotene on the Incidence of Lung Cancer and Other Cancers in Male Smokers." Heinonen, O.P. and Albanes. D. *New England Journal of Medicine*, vol. 330, Apr. 14, 1994, pp. l029–35.

"Elderly Subjects Aged 70 Years and Above Have Different Risk Factors of Ischaemic and Heomorrhagic Strokes Compared to Younger Subjects." Woo, O. et al. *Journal of American Geriatrics Society*, Feb. 1991.

Felmore Guide to the Menopause. Stewart, M. Women's Nutritional Advice Service, P.O. Box 268, Hove, East Sussex BN3 1RW.

Fish Foundation Research Update, June 1993.

Fish Foundation News Update, reporting Dr. Jill. Belch at 3rd International Congress on Essential Polyunsaturates and Eicosanoids, Adelaide, Australia, Mar. 1993.

"Fish Oil—More than a Red Herring?" Rice, R. *Practice Nurse*, vol. 4, no. 3, 1991, pp. l43–45.

"Fish Oil Reduces Blood Pressure." *What Doctors Don't Tell You*, vol. 4, no. 7.

"Food Carbohydrates—The Australian Connection." *Dietary Fiber*, vol. 1, no. 2, 1993, pp. 25–48.

"Further Evidence of Heart Benefit of Red Wine." *Pulse*, Mar. 26, 1994.

"Garlic: A Review of its Relationship to Malignant Disease." Dausch, J. and Nixon, D.W. *Preventative Medicine*, vol. 19, 1990, pp. 346–61.

"Garlic, Onions and Cardiovascular Risk Factors. A Review of the Evidence from Human Experiments." Kleijnen, J. et al. *British Journal of Clinical Pharmacology*, vol. 28, 1989, pp. 535–44.

"How to Avoid Osteoporosis." Chaitow, Leon. *Here's Health*, Mar. 1992.

"The Importance of Magnesium in the Management of Primary Postmenopausal Osteoporosis." Abraham, G. *Journal of Nutritional Medicine*, vol. 2, 1991, pp. 165–78.

In Search of the Secrets of Aging. National Institute on Aging, Dept. of Health and Human Services, May 1993, National Institutes of Health pub. no. 93-2756.

"Kervran's Silica." Kenton, L. Leaflet from Health Innovations, based on proceedings from Halsoprodukter Silica Symposium, Paris, 1988.

"Live Twice as Long, Age Half as Fast." Poppy, J. *Longevity*, Oct. 1993.

"Low Serum Cholesterol Concentrations and Short Term Mortality from Injuries in Men and Women." Lindberg, G. et al. *British Medical Journal*, vol. 305, Aug. 1, 1992.

"Mediterranean Alpha-Linolenic Acid-Rich Diet in Secondary Prevention of Coronary Heart Disease." Lorgeril, M. de et al. *Lancet*, vol. 343, June 11, 1994.

"Mighty Vitamins." Skerrett, P.J. *Medical World News*, vol. 34, no. 1, Jan. 1993.

"Mind the Quacks!" Lobstein, T. *The Food Magazine*, Feb./Apr. 1993.

"National Osteoporosis Society Calls for Urgent Review of Recommended Daily Calcium Intake." National Osteoporosis Society press release, Aug. 1993.

"Nibbling Versus Gorging: Metabolic Advantages of Increased Meal Frequency." Jenkins, D. et al. *New England Journal of Medicine*, vol. 321, no. 14, pp. 929–33.

Normal Human Aging: The Baltimore Longitudinal Study of Aging. Shock, N.W. et al. U.S. Government Printing Office, 1984.

The Nutrition of Elderly People. Department of Health HMSO, 1992.

"Nutrition Intervention Trials in Linxian, China." Blot, W.J. *Journal of the National Cancer Institute*, vol. 85, no. 18, Sept. 15, 1993.

"Perk or Poison?" Greener, M. *Nursing Times*, vol. 89, no. 49, Dec. 8, 1993.

"Plasma Antioxidants, Indices of Lipid Peroxidation and Coronary Heart Disease Risk Factors in a Scottish Population." Duthie, G. *Nutrition Research*, vol. 12, supplement 1, 1992.

"Preservatives May Help Fight Cancer." News release, Imperial Cancer Research Fund, Apr. 1994.

"A Prospective Study of Alcohol Consumption and Bone Mineral Density." Holbrook, T. and Barrett-Connor, E. *British Medical Journal*, vol. 306, June 5, 1993.

"Relation of Smoking and Low-to-Moderate Alcohol Consumption to Change in Cognitive Function." Hebert, L. E. et al. *American Journal of Epidemiology*, vol. 137, no. 8, pp. 881–91.

"Risk of Death from Cancer and Ischaemic Heart Disease in Meat and Non-Meat Eaters." Thorogood, M. et al. *British Medical Journal*, vol. 308, June 25, 1994.

Satiety and Dietary Fibre: Comparison of Breakfasts Containing Soluble and Insoluble Fibre. Delargy, H.J. et al. BioPsychology Group, University of Leeds, 1993.

"A Screening and Counselling Program for Prevention of Osteoporosis." Gutin, B. et al. *Osteoporosis International*, vol. 2, no. 5, Sept. 1992, pp. 252–56.

"Serum Antioxidant Vitamins and Risk of Cataract." Knekt, H. et al. *British Medical Journal*, Dec. 5, 1992.

"A Study of the Effects of Bifidus on Intestinal Transit Time." Grimaud, J. C. et al. Report supported by Gervais-Danone, Sept. 1, 1992.

"A Total Dietary Program Emphasizing Magnesium and Calcium." Abraham, G. and Grewal, H. *Journal of Reproductive Medicine*, vol. 35, no. 5, May 5, 1990, pp. 503–7.

"Unsaturated vs. Saturated Fats." Family Heart Association fact sheet, no. 4.

"Vitamin C Depletion and Pressure Sores in Elderly Patients with Femoral Neck Fractures." Goode, H. et al. *British Medical Journal*, vol. 305, Oct. 17, 1992.

"Vitamin D and Calcium to Prevent Hip Fractures in Elderly Women." Chapuy, M.C. et al. *New England Journal of Medicine*, vol. 327, Dec. 3, 1992, pp. 1637–42.

"Vitamin E Consumption and the Risk of Coronary Heart Disease in Women." Stampfer, M.J. et al. *New England Journal of Medicine*, May 20, 1993.

"Vitamin E Research Summary." *Veris*, Jan. 1993.

"Vitamins Get a New Lease of Life." Hawkes, N. *The Times*, June 3, 1993.

Your Good Health: The Medicinal Benefits of Wine Drinking. Maury, E. Souvenir Press, London, 1993.

THE CHALLENGE OF STAYING HEALTHY

"Ageing and Drug Metabolism." Woodhouse, K. Research Into Ageing briefing, Sept. 16, 1993.

Ageing: The Facts. Coni, N. et al. Oxford University Press, 1992.

Ageless Ageing. Kenton, L. Century, 1985.

"Alzheimer's Disease." Levy, R. Research Into Ageing briefing, May 1993.

"Arthritis." FDA consumer reprint, July 1991.

"The Aspirin Papers." Underwood, M. J. and More, R.S. *British Medical Journal*, vol. 308, Jan. 8, 1994.

"Beneficial Effect of Oestrogen on Exercise-Induced Myocardial Ischaemia in Women with Coronary Artery Disease." Rosano, M.C.G. et al. *Lancet*, vol. 342, July 17, 1993.

"Bone Scan Case Fails for Lack of Evidence." Report from Leeds University School of Public Health, *Hospital Doctor*, Jan. 9, 1992.

Cancer Tests You Should Know About—A Guide for People 65 and Over, National Institutes of Health, pub. no. 93-3256.

"The Carnegie Inquiry on Health: Ability and Wellbeing in the Third Age." Research paper no. 9, 1992.

"Cause for Caution on Cholesterol Care." *Hospital Doctor*, June 10, 1993.

"CHD in Women: Discrimination is Needed." Swan, J. and Stevenson, J. *Geriatric Medicine*, Jan. 1993.

Cholesterol and Health 33, newsletter of the Family Heart Association, Autumn 1993.

"Cholesterol Levels at Which Drug Treatment Should be Considered." British Heart Foundation statement, July 1993.

"Effect of Aspirin and Non-Steroidal Anti-Inflammatory Drugs on Colorectal Adenomas: Case-Control Study of Subjects Participating in Nottingham Faecal Occult Blood Screening Programme." Logan, R.F.A. et al. *British Medical Journal*, vol. 307, July 31, 1993.

"Effects of Human Growth Hormone in Men over 60 Years Old." Rudman, D. et al. *New England Journal of Medicine*, vol. 323, 1990, pp. 1–6.

"The Effect of Postmenopausal Estrogen Therapy on Bone Density In Elderly Women." Felson, D. T. et al. *New England Journal of Medicine*, vol. 329, Oct. 14, 1993.

"Eye Openers." *Here's Health*, Apr. 1993.

"The Eyes Have It." Research into Ageing press information, Oct. 15, 1993.

"The Foetal and Infant Origins of Ageing." Barker, D. Research Into Ageing briefing, July 1, 1992.

"Foot Problems of the Elderly." *Geriatric Medicine*, Jan. 1991.

"Gastroenterology Seminar on Colorectal Management." *Hospital Update*, Dec. 1991.

A Gene for Atherosclerosis. Dawson, S. Research Into Ageing briefing, 1991.

"Gene Jolt." *Longevity*, Aug. 1993.

"Gene Therapy Begins." Davies, K. and Williamson, B. *British Medical Journal*, vol. 306, June 19, 1993.

Health and Healthy Living: A Guide for Older People. Department of Health, Nov. 1991.

Health Survey for England. Department of Health, 1991.

"Heart Disease Study Invokes Memories of Leningrad Siege." Radford, T. *The Times*, July 26, 1993.

"Eye Care." Help the Aged leaflet.

"Fitter Feet." Help the Aged leaflet.

"Hormone Replacement Therapy and Heart Disease." British Heart Foundation statement, July 5, 1993.

"How Can Doctors Diagnose Colorectal Cancer Earlier?" Maclennan, I. and Hill, J. *British Medical Journal*, vol. 306, June 26, 1993.

Human Aging and Later Life, ed. A.M. Warner, Edward Arnold, 1989.

"Immunisation Against Influenza Among People Aged Over 65 Living at Home in Leicestershire During Winter 1991–2." Nicholson, K. G. *British Medical Journal*, vol. 306, Apr. 10, 1993.

"The Influence of Age on Policies for Admission and Thrombolysis in Coronary Care Units in the U.K." Dudley, N.J. and Burns, E. *Age and Ageing*, vol. 21, 1992, pp. 95–102.

"Influenza Vaccination: Your View." *Geriatric Medicine*, Nov. 1992.

"In Healthy Fashion." Report on trainers, *Upbeat* (BUPA magazine), Jan. 1994.

In Search of the Secrets of Aging. National Institute on Aging, Department of Health and Human Services, May 1993, National Institutes of Health pub. no. 93-2756.

"Is the Serum Cholesterol-Coronary Heart Disease Relationship Modified by Activity Level in Older Persons?" Harris, T. et al. *Journal of the American Geriatrics Society*, vol. 3, 1991, pp. 747–54.

Life Extension Report on Biomarkers. American Academy of Anti-Aging Medicine, Nov. 1993.

"Management Guidelines in Essential Hypertension: Report of the Second Working Party of the British Hypertension Society." Sever, P. et al. *British Medical Journal*, vol. 306, April 1993.

"Medical Management of Prostate Cancer." Gallagher, C. J. *Geriatric Medicine*, Feb. 1992.

Menopause. National Institute on Aging, Dec. 1992.

The Menopause—Risks and Side-Effects of HRT. Cust, M. et al. Focus International Monograph Series, Medicom, 1989.

"Muscle Weakness in Women Occurs at an Earlier Age Than in Men, But Strength is Preserved by Hormone Replacement Therapy." Phillips, S.K. et al. *Clinical Science*, vol. 84, 1993, pp. 95–98.

The New Approach to Osteoporosis: A Guide for General Practitioners. National Osteoporosis Society, 1990.

Osteoporosis and the Risk of Fracture. Office of Health Economics, 1990.

"Osteoporosis in the 1990s (2): Prevention and Management." Garton, M. J. and Reid, D. M. *Hospital Update*, July 1993, pp. 412–17.

"Pelvic Muscle Exercise for Stress Urinary Incontinence in Elderly Women." Wells, T. J. et al. *Journal of the American Geriatrics Society*, vol. 39, 1991, pp. 785–91.

"Postmenopausal Estrogen Therapy and Cardiovascular Disease: Ten-Year Follow-Up from the Nurses Health Study." Stampfer, M. J. et al. *New England Journal of Medicine*, vol. 325, no. 11, 1991, pp. 756–62.

"Prevalence Screening for Ovarian Cancer in Postmenopausal Women." Jacobs, I. et al. *British Medical Journal*, vol. 306, Apr. 17, 1993.

Progress Report on Alzheimer's Disease. National Institute on Aging, pub. no. 92-3409, 1992.

"Rationale for Primary Prevention Study Using Low-Dose Aspirin to Prevent Coronary and Cerebrovascular Disease of the Elderly." Silagy, C.A. et al. *Journal of the American Geriatrics Society*, vol. 39, May 1991.

"Rationale for Stopping Cervical Screening in Women Over 50." Van Wijn-gaarden, W. J. and Duncan, I.D. *British Medical Journal*, vol. 306, Apr. 10, 993.

"Recent Advances in Alzheimer's Disease." Rosser, M. Research Into Ageing briefing, Dec. 1993.

"Regaining Lost Hearing." *Longevity*, Aug. 1993.

"Relation of Fingerprints and Shape of the Palm to Fetal Growth and Adult Blood Pressure." Godfrey, K.M. et al. *British Medical Journal*, vol. 307, Aug. 14, 1993.

"Relation of Helicobacter Pylori Infection and Coronary Heart Disease." Mendall, M. A. et al. *British Heart Journal*, vol. 71, 1994, pp. 437–39.

"Relation of Infant Feeding to Adult Serum Cholesterol Concentration and Death from Ischaemic Heart Disease." Fall, C.H.D. et al. *British Medical Journal*, vol. 304, March 28, 1992.

"The Relation of Small Head Circumference and Thinness at Birth to Death from Cardiovascular Disease in Adult Life." Barker, D. J. P. et al. *British Medical Journal*, vol. 306, Feb. 13, 1993.

"Researchers Call for Regular Screening for Women at High Risk of Ovarian Cancer." Press release from Imperial Cancer Research Fund, Apr. 17, 1993.

"Researchers Take Genetic Clue to Heart." Pinn, S. *Hospital Doctor*, Mar. 4, 1993.

"The Risks of High Cholesterol and Elderly People." *Geriatric Medicine*, Mar. 1991.

"Shoe Sole Thickness and Hardness Influence Balance in Older Men." Robbins, S. et al. *Journal of the American Geriatrics Society*, vol. 40, 1992, pp. 1089–94.

"Silicon and the Bioavailability of Aluminium—Nutritional Aspects." Birchall, J. D. Food, *Nutrition and Chemical Toxicity*, Smith-Gordon, 1993.

Special Report on Aging. National Institute on Aging, pub. no. 92-3409, 1992.

"Study Fuels Row on Breast Tests for the Under-50." *Hospital Door*, Oct. 29, 1992.

"Tamoxifen Reduces Bone Loss in Women with Breast Cancer." Mazess, R. et al. Paper presented at the American Society for Bone and Mineral Research, Aug. 1990.

"Towards Gene Therapy for Malignant Melanoma." Press release from Imperial Cancer Research Fund, Mar. 1993.

"Tracing the Real Cause of Disease." Wolff, S. Research Into Ageing report, Oct. 1992.

"The Triglyceride Issue: A View from Framingham." Castelli, W. *American Heart Journal*, Aug. 1986, pp. 432–37.

"Viropause: A Syndrome of Testosterone Resistance Associated with Premature Ageing in Men" and "Testosterone Treatment of the Male Menopause or Male Viropause." Carruthers, M. unpublished papers.

"When Do you Need an Antacid?" FDA consumer reprint, May 1993.

"Where are the Women in Studies of Coronary Heart Disease?" Khaw, K. *British Medical Journal*, vol. 306, May 1, 1993.

Who? What? Where? Resources for Women's Health and Aging. National Institutes of Health, pub. no. 91-323, Mar. 1992.

"Why Menopause?" Rogers, A. *Evolutionary Ecology*, vol. 7, 1993, pp. 406–20.

"You Are What They Ate." Hawkes, N. *The Times Saturday* Review, June 6, 1992.

THE CHALLENGE OF LOOKING GOOD

"Associations of Abdominal Adiposity, Fasting Insulin, Sex Hormone Binding Globulin, and Estrone with Lipids and Lipoproteins in Post-Menopausal Women." Folsom, A.R. et al. *Atherosclerosis*, vol. 79, 1989, pp. 21–27.

"Body Image, Attitudes to Weight, and Misperceptions of Figure Preferences of the Opposite Sex: A Comparison of Men and Women in Two Generations." Rozin, P. and Fallon, A. *Journal of Abnormal Psychology*, vol. 97, no. 3, pp. 342–45.

"Cellex-C™ in Search of Youth." Press release issued by Lorraine Meisner, University of Wisconsin, Madison.

"Effect of Very Low Calorie Diet on Body Composition and Exercise Response in Sedentary Women." Eston, R. G. et al. *European Journal of Applied Physiology and Occupational Physiology*, vol. 65, no. 5, 1992, pp. 452–58.

"Fat Chance for Diets in the Serotonin Trap." *Hospital Doctor*, Nov. 19, 1992.

"An FDA Guide to Dieting." Papazian, R. Quoting *New England Journal of Medicine* research on identical twins, Sept. 1993.

"Female and Male Perceptions of Ideal Body Shapes." Cohn, L. D. and Alder, N. E. *Psychology of Women Quarterly*, vol. 16, 1992, pp. 69–79.

"Hazard of Obesity: The Framingham Experience." Higgins, M. et al. Acta-Med-Scand 223/suppl. 723, 1988, pp. 23–36.

"Lines Lead to Deep-Sea Tablets." Hawkes, N. *The Times*, Mar. 9, 1993.

"Men's Skin Stays Young as Women Wrinkle." *GP Magazine*, Apr. 1993.

"Obesity as an Independent Risk Factor for Cardiovascular Disease: A 26-year Follow-Up of Participants in the Framingham Heart Study." Hubert, H. B. et al. *Circulation*, vol. 67, no. 5, 1983, pp. 968–77.

"Past, Present and Future, Ageing and Longevity." Vidik, A. *European Journal of Gerontology*, Sept. 91.

"Petroleum Jelly's Anti-Aging Surprises." *Longevity*, Dec. 1992.

Physical Activity, Aging and Sports, vol. 1, ed. Harris, R. and Harris, S. Center for the Study of Aging, Albany NY.

"A Prospective Study of Obesity and Risk of Coronary Heart Disease in Women." Manson, J. E. et al. *New England Journal of Medicine*, vol. 322, 1990, pp. 882–89.

"Psychological and Behavioral Differences Among Females Classified as Bulimic, Obligatory Exerciser and Normal Control." Krejcietal, R. C. *Psychiatry*, vol. 55, no. 2, May 1992, pp. 185–93.

"Variability of Body Weight and Health Outcomes in the Framingham Population." Lissner, L. et al. *New England Journal of Medicine*, vol. 324, June 27, 1991, pp. 1839–44.

"Whole Body Calorimetry in Man and Animals." Dauncey, M.J. *Thermochimica Acta*, vol. 193, pp. 1–40, Elsevier, 1991.

THE BRAIN CHALLENGE

"Age Associated Memory Impairment." *British Medical Journal*, vol. 304, Jan. 4, 1992.

Ageing: The Facts. Coni, N. et al. Oxford University Press, 1992.

"Age-Related Changes in Memory." Huppert, F. A. in *Handbook of Neurology*, ed. Boller, F. and Grafman, J. Elsevier, 1988.

"Depression in the Elderly." Guidelines from the Royal College of Psychiatrists, Apr. 1993.

"Do Alcoholics Drink Their Neurons Away?" Jensen, G. B. *Lancet*, vol. 342, Nov. 12, 1993.

"The Effect of Age on Driving Skills." Carr, D. et al. *Journal of American Geriatrics Society*, vol. 40, 1992, pp. 567–73.

"Exercise for Older Women: A Training Method and Its Influences on Physical and Cognitive Performance." Hassmen, P. et al. *European Journal of Applied Physiology*, vol. 64, 1992, pp. 460–66.

"Explanatory Style and Cell-Mediated Immunity in Elderly Men and Women." Rodin, J. et al. *Health Psychology* vol. 10, no. 4, 1991, pp. 229–235.

"Gender Differences in Depression: Historical Changes." Silverstein, B. and Perlick, D. *Acta Psychiatrica Scandinavia*, vol. 84. no. 4, Oct. 1991, pp. 327–31.

"Ginkgo biloba." Kleijnen, J. and Knipschild, P. *Lancet*, vol. 340, Nov. 7, 1992.

"How the Mind Ages." *Psychology Today*, Nov./Dec. 1993.

"Hypertension Affects Neurobehavioral Functioning." Blumenthal, J.A. et al. *Psychosomatic Medicine*, vol. 55, no. 1, Jan./Feb. 1993, pp. 44–50.

"Influence of Mood on Judgements About Health and Illness." Salovey, P. et al. *Emotional and Social Judgements*, ed. Forgas, J. Pergamon Press, 1991.

"Long-Term Alcohol Intake and Cognition in Aging Twins." Christian, J.C. et al. Report presented at the Research Society on Alcoholism annual meeting, 1993.

"Low Systolic Blood Pressure and Self-Perceived Wellbeing in Middle-Aged Men." Rosengren, A. et al. *British Medical Journal*, vol. 306, Jan. 23, 1993.

"Napping and 24-Hour Sleep/Wake Patterns in Healthy Elderly and Young Adults," Buysse, D. J. et al. *Journal of the American Geriatrics Society*, vol. 40, 1992, pp. 779–86.

"The Nightmare of Ageing." Press release from Age Concern, Jan. 1992.

"A Patient with Severe Iron-Deficiency Anaemia and Memory Disturbance." Anezaki, T. et al. *Internal Medicine*, vol. 31, no. 11, Nov. 1992.

"Plain Talk about Depression." National Institute of Mental Health, Apr. 1993.

"The Potential of the Ageing Brain for Structural Regeneration." Diamond, M. In *Recent Advances of Psychogeriatrics*, ed. Arie, T. Churchill Livingstone, 1985.

"Psychology and Survival." Phillips, D. P. et al. *Lancet*, vol. 342, Nov. 6, 1993.

"The Relationship Between Diet and Mental Health." Cook, R. and Benton, D. *Personality and Individual Differences*, vol. 14, no. 3, 1993, pp. 397–403.

"A Scale of Measuring the Occurrence of Positive States of Mind: A Preliminary Report," Horowitz, M. et al. *Psychosomatic Medicine*, vol. 50, 1988, pp. 477–83.

"Self-Assessed Job Satisfaction and Ischaemic Heart Disease Mortality: A Ten-Year Follow-Up of Urban Bus Drivers." Nettersllam, B. *International Journal of Epidemiology*, vol. 22, no. 1, 1993, pp. 51–56.

"Sleep and Sleep Problems in Elderly People." Swift, C. G. and Shapiro, C. M. *British Medical Journal*, vol. 306, May 29, 1993.

"The Sleep Apnoea/Hypopnoea Syndrome and Snoring." Douglas, N. J. *British Medical Journal*, vol. 306, Apr. 17, 1993.

SSRIs "Set for Frontline Role in Depression," *Hospital Doctor*, June 10, 1993.

"Stay-Young Drugs." Lawren, B. *Longevity*, Sept. 1993.

"Stressful Life Events, Social Support, and Mortality in Men Born in 1933." Rosengren, A. et al. *British Medical Journal*, vol. 307, Oct. 30, 1993.

"Usefulness of Commercial Memory Aids As a Function of Age." Petro, S. J. et al. *International Journal of Aging and Human Development*, vol. 33, no. 4, 1991, pp. 295–309.

Which? Way to Health, Feb. 1993.

THE LIFESTYLE CHALLENGE

"Age and Attitudes: Main Results from a Eurobarometer Survey." Commission of the European Communities, 1993.

Age Barriers at Work. Itzin, C. and Phillipson, C. Metropolitan Authorities Recruitment Agency, 1993.

"Age Is No Bar to Sexually Acquired Infection." Rogstad, K. and Bignell, C. J. *Age and Ageing*, Sept. 1991.

Ageless Body, Timeless Mind. Chopra, D. Rider 1993.

"The British Gas Report on Attitudes to Ageing." 1991.

"Flexible Working is Here to Stay." Institute of Management press release, Sept. 1994.

The Fountain of Age. Friedan, B. Simon and Schuster, 1993.

Gender and Later Life. Arber, S. and Ginn, J. Sage 1991.

"The Great Symphony Orchestra—A Relatively Good Place to Grow Old." Smith, D. W. E. International Journal of Aging and Human Development, vol. 27, no. 4, 1988, pp. 233–46.

"A Growing Number of Elders Live Alone and Prefer It." *AARP Bulletin*, Sept. 1993.

Individual Quality of Life in the Healthy Elderly. Browne, J.P. et al. Royal College of Surgeons in Ireland, Dublin, 1994.

The Janus Report. Wiley, 1993.

"The Long-Term Marriage: Perceptions of Stability and Satisfaction." Lauer, R.H. et al. *International Journal of Aging and Development*, vol. 31, no. 3, 1990, pp. 189–95.

"Marital Coital Activity in Men at the Age of 75: Relation to Somatic, Psychiatric and Social Factors at the Age of 70." Persson, G. and Svanborg, A. *Journal of the American Geriatrics Society*, vol. 40, 1992, pp. 439–44.

"Midlife Myths." Gallagher, W. *Atlantic Monthly*, May 1993.

MIDMAC Program, The John D. and Catherine T. MacArthur Foundation.

"Predicates of Personal Control Among Middle Aged and Young Old Men and Women in Middle America." Huyck, M. Hellie. *International Journal of Aging and Human Development*, vol. 32, no. 4, 1991, pp. 261–275.

A Profile of Older Americans: 1995. Program Resources Dept., American Association of Retired Persons and the Administration on Aging, U.S. Dept. of Health and Human Services, 1995.

"The Quality of Older Life." *New York Times*, Nov. 6, 1993.

"Sex In Later Life." MORI poll, 1993.

"Successful Ageing and Life Course Reciprocity." Antonucci, T. and Jackson, J. Institute for Social Research, University of Michigan, Ann Arbor, Michigan.

Third Age Lifestyles, Mintel, 1993.

Turning the Pages: Sexuality Across the Life Course. Rossi, A. University of Chicago Press 1994.

"Youthful Ideas About Old Age." Falchikov, *International Journal of Aging and Health Development*, vol. 3,1 no. 2, 1990.

Index

About the Author

Helen Franks is a journalist and an author who has contributed to leading newspapers and magazines on health matters and social issues, including aging and the elderly. Her books include *Prime Time*, a study of women in midlife, and *Bone Boosters—Natural Ways to Beat Osteoporosis* (with Diana Moran). She lives in London and is married with three children and one grandchild. She walks, practices yoga and tap dances to keep fit.

Ulysses Press Health Books

AFTER THE DIAGNOSIS
Joann LeMaistre, Ph.D.

> With the diagnosis of a chronic illness comes a blow to the psyche that can be as devastating as the symptoms. This book, written by a psychologist who has multiple sclerosis, explains how chronically ill people can be able-hearted when it is no longer possible to be able-bound. $12.95

THE BOOK OF KOMBUCHA
Beth Ann Petro

> *The Book of Kombucha* cuts through the hype to answer all the questions and concerns surrounding kombucha, one of America's fastest growing alternative health treatments. Drawing on the most up-to-date research, the book gives detailed instructions on how to obtain, brew and use kombucha. $11.95

COUNT OUT CHOLESTEROL
Art Ulene, M.D. and Val Ulene, M.D.

> Complete with counter and detailed dietary plan, this companion resource to the *Count Out Cholesterol Cookbook* shows how to design a cholesterol-lowering program that's right for you. $12.95
> *Count Out Cholesterol Cookbook*, $14.95

IRRITABLE BOWEL SYNDROME:
A NATURAL APPROACH
Rosemary Nicol

> This book offers a natural approach to a problem millions of sufferers have. The author clearly defines the symptoms and offers a dietary and stress-reduction program for relieving the effects of this disease. $9.95

KNOW YOUR BODY: THE ATLAS OF ANATOMY
Introduction by Trevor Weston, M.D.

> Designed to provide a comprehensive and concise guide to the structure of the human body, *Know Your Body* offers more than 250 color illustrations. An easy-to-follow road map of the human body. $12.95

LAST WISHES: A HANDBOOK TO GUIDE YOUR SURVIVORS
Lucinda Page Knox, M.S.W. and Michael D. Knox, Ph.D.

> A simple do-it-yourself workbook, *Last Wishes* helps people put their affairs in order and eases the burden on survivors. It allows them to plan their own funeral and leave final instructions for survivors. $12.95

LOSE WEIGHT WITH DR. ART ULENE
Art Ulene, M.D.

> This best-selling weight-loss book offers a 28-day program for taking off the pounds and keeping them off forever. $12.95

MOOD FOODS
Dr. William Vayda

> *Mood Foods* shows how the foods you eat can influence your emotions, behavior and personality. It also explains how a proper diet can help to alleviate such common complaints as PMS, hyperactivity, mood swings and stress. $9.95

PANIC ATTACKS: A NATURAL APPROACH
Shirley Trickett

> Addresses the problem of panic attacks using a holistic approach. Focusing on diet and relaxation, the book helps you prevent future attacks. $8.95

SECRETS OF SEXUAL BODY LANGUAGE
Martin Lloyd-Elliott

> This book unlocks the secret messages and sexual implications of body language. It shows how to use nonverbal communication to understand the sexual intentions of others and to send messages that properly convey one's true feelings. $16.95

THE VITAMIN STRATEGY
Art Ulene, M.D. and Val Ulene, M.D.

> A game plan for good health, this book helps readers design a vitamin and mineral program tailored to their individual needs. $11.95

YOUR NATURAL PREGNANCY: A GUIDE TO COMPLEMENTARY THERAPIES
Anne Charlish

> This timely book brings together the many complementary therapies such as aromatherapy, massage, homeopathy, acupressure, herbal medicine and meditation, that can benefit pregnant women. $16.95

To order these or other Ulysses Press books, fill out the order form on the next page, or contact Ulysses Press at 800-377-2542 (P.O. Box 3440, Berkeley, CA 94703-3440). All retail orders are shipped free of charge. California residents must include sales tax. Allow two to three weeks for delivery.

Order Form

Ulysses Press books are available at bookstores everywhere. If any of the following titles are unavailable at your local bookstore, ask the bookseller to order them. Or you can order them directly from Ulysses Press.

_____*After the Diagnosis*, $12.95
_____*The Book of Kombucha*, $11.95
_____*Count Out Cholesterol*, $12.95
_____*Count Out Cholesterol Cookbook*, $14.95
_____*Irritable Bowel Syndrome: A Natural Approach*, $9.95
_____*Know Your Body: The Atlas of Anatomy*, $12.95
_____*Last Wishes: A Handbook to Guide Your Survivors*, $12.95
_____*Lose Weight with Dr. Art Ulene*, $12.95
_____*Mood Foods*, $9.95
_____*Panic Attacks: A Natural Approach*, $8.95
_____*Secrets of Sexual Body Language*, $16.95
_____*The Vitamin Strategy*, $11.95
_____*Your Natural Pregnancy: A Guide to Complementary Therapies*, $16.95

Mark the book(s) you're ordering and enter the total cost here 🠾 [＿＿＿＿]

California residents add 8% sales tax here 🠾 [＿＿＿＿]

Shipping, check box for your preferred method and enter cost here 🠾 [＿＿＿＿]

❑ BOOK RATE   **FREE! FREE! FREE!**

❑ PRIORITY MAIL $3.00 First book, $1.00/each additional book

❑ UPS 2-DAY AIR $7.00 First book, $1.00/each additional book

Billing, enter total amount due here and check method of payment 🠾 [＿＿＿＿]

❑ CHECK   ❑ MONEY ORDER   ❑ VISA/MASTERCARD

NAME_____PHONE _____

ADDRESS_____

_____

CITY _____ STATE _____ ZIP _____

MONEY-BACK GUARANTEE ON DIRECT ORDERS PLACED THROUGH ULYSSES PRESS.